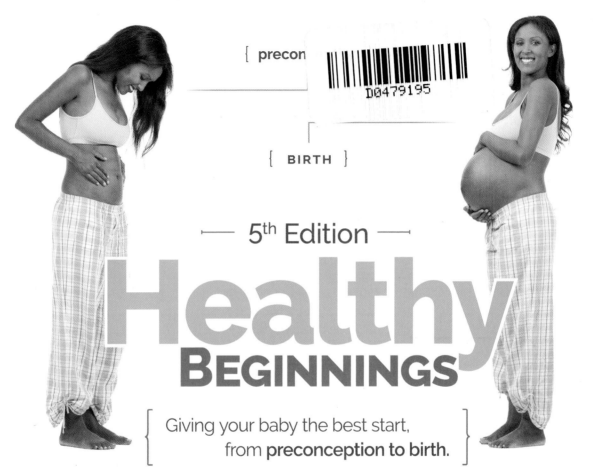

{ preconc

{ BIRTH }

— 5ᵗʰ Edition —

Healthy
BEGINNINGS

{ Giving your baby the best start,
from **preconception to birth**. }

Principal Author: Nan Schuurmans, MD, FRCSC; Edmonton, AB
Editor: Jennifer Blake, MD, FRCSC; Chief Executive Officer, SOGC; Ottawa, ON

WILEY

ISBN 9781119283973 (Paperback)
ISBN 9781119283980 (ePDF)
Cover Design: Wiley
Cover Images: © aleksandarvelasevic/Getty Images, Inc., © RuslanDashinsky/Getty Images, Inc.
Designed by: Red Wagon Studio
Illustrations: Julie Dorion

Printed in the United States of America

10 9 8 7 6 5 4 3 2 1

Contents

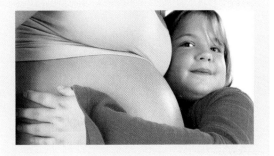

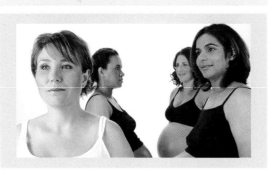

CHAPTER THREE
Gentle growth: the second trimester 87

CHAPTER FOUR
The home stretch: the third trimester 107

Acknowledgements

Healthy Beginnings: Giving your baby the best start, from preconception to birth, fifth edition, is based on the Society of Obstetricians and Gynaecologists' clinical practice guidelines.

The Society of Obstetricians and Gynaecologists of Canada would like to thank the following organizations and individuals for sharing their experience and knowledge:

Best Start Resource Centre
Canadian Paediatric Society
Central South West Reproductive Health Working Group
Champlain Maternal Newborn Regional Program: Christina Cantin, RN,
    MScN, PNC(C), Perinatal Consultant
Kathy Chan, RN, BScN, IBCLC, Public Health Nurse
City of Hamilton Public Health Department, Family Health Division—
    Breastfeeding Resource Team: Dana Haas, RN, BScN, IBCLC, Public
    Health Nurse/Lactation Consultant
Jocelynn Cook, PhD
E. Laura Cruz, MD, CCFP(SEM), Dip. Sport Med
Dad Central Ontario: Brian Russell, Provincial Coordinator
Fraser Health, British Columbia: Sidney Harper, Baby Friendly Initiative
    Lead
Susan Gallagher, RN, BScN, Public Health Nurse
Edna Marie Grajales, RN, BScN, Public Health Nurse
Édith Guilbert, MD, MSc, FCFP
Hastings Prince Edward Public Health: Jessica Richardson, Registered
    Dietitian
Immunize Canada: Lucie Marisa Bucci, Senior Manager
Jennifer Jocko, MD, FRCSC
KFL&A Public Health: Darlene Johnson, Public Health Nurse
Marg La Salle, RN, BScN, IBCLC, CCHN and BFI lead assessor
Lisa Morgan, RM, MA, PhD (candidate)
Motherisk Program
Jack Newman, MD
Ontario Public Health Association's (OPHA) Reproductive Health
    Workgroup

Ontario Society of Nutrition Professionals in Public Health (OSNPPH)

Andrea Page's Original Fitmom

Parachute: Pamela Fuselli, VP, Knowledge Transfer & Stakeholder Relations

Physical Activity Resource Centre (PARC), managed by Ophea

Provincial Council for Maternal and Child Health—Maternal Newborn Advisory Committee

Matthuschka Sheedy, RN, BNSc, ICCE

Simcoe Muskoka District Health Unit: Becky Blair, RD

St. Joseph's Health Centre: Alice Ordean, MD, CCFP, MHSc, FCFP, DABAM, Associate Professor, Department of Family & Community Medicine; Medical Director, Toronto Centre for Substance Use in Pregnancy

Swati Scott, RD, IBCLC

Toronto Public Health: Catriona Mill, RN, MHSc, CCHN(c), Chair, OPHA Reproductive Health Workgroup & Health Promotion Specialist

University of Ottawa Heart Institute: Andrew Pipe, CM, MD, LLD(Hon), DSc(Hon), Chief, Division of Prevention & Rehabilitation

Evelyn Vaccari, MHSc, RD, Consultant Nutrition Promotion

Sandra Walker, SSW, BSW

R. Douglas Wilson, MD, MSc

Special thanks to all who have contributed on previous editions of this publication and a special acknowledgement to Vyta Senikas, MDCM, FRCSC, and André B. Lalonde, MD, FRCSC.

Foreword

Pregnancy is a special time in a woman's life as she prepares for the life-changing event of adding a new member to the family. The fifth edition of *Healthy Beginnings* was revised by the Society of Obstetricians and Gynaecologists of Canada to help bring women the latest information to help them have healthy pregnancies.

This handbook is for women with low-risk pregnancies—about 90% of all pregnancies in Canada. Reducing risk is a key part of having a healthy pregnancy. In this new edition of the handbook, we place greater emphasis on preconception—the time just before the baby is conceived—and also on early pregnancy—the first 3 months after conception.

The advice and information in *Healthy Beginnings* is evidence-based. This means that the content reflects current knowledge and comes from the latest proven research and professional practices in Canada. The guidelines contained in this handbook for care before pregnancy, during pregnancy, and after the birth have been updated and have been reviewed by numerous experts including obstetricians, midwives, many doctors and nurses. The information should not be seen as an exclusive course of treatment or procedure to be followed. Your health care provider should be consulted and will advise you on your pregnancy and/or specific concerns.

International research shows that if pregnant women are aware of how their bodies prepare for birth and what their growing babies need, they will have healthier pregnancies, and more babies will be born full-size, full-term, and healthy.

Healthy Beginnings provides you with the information you need to make healthy choices during your pregnancy. It serves as a notebook where you can record the details of your pregnancy, prenatal visits, and your birth experience. Forms are included where you can gather important information you will need during your pregnancy. Space has been provided at the end of each chapter for you to write out questions for your next appointments. Record the changes in your body and your feelings for reference at your next appointment or even months and years later, when your notes will remind you of this special time.

Enjoy your pregnancy and look forward to meeting your baby!

Dr. Nan Schuurmans, MD, FRCSC

Notes to the reader:

In this handbook, the words *he* and *she* are used equally. The term *health care provider* refers to specialists, obstetricians, gynaecologists, family physicians, nurses, midwives, and other health care practitioners.

The Baby-Friendly Initiative (BFI) is a program of the World Health Organization and UNICEF to increase hospital and community support for promoting, supporting, and protecting breastfeeding. Every effort has been made to ensure the content of the fifth edition of *Healthy Beginnings* complies with the requirements of the Baby-Friendly Initiative and meets the BFI 10 Steps Practice Outcome Indicators for Hospitals and Community Health Services. For more information go to www.breastfeedingcanada.ca/BFI.aspx.

The Society of Obstetricians and Gynaecologists of Canada (SOGC) is a long-standing professional society with a growing and robust membership that consist of over 3,500 obstetricians, gynaecologists, family physicians, nurses, midwives, researchers, and trainees. The mission of the SOGC is to promote excellence in the practice of obstetrics and gynaecology and to advance the health of women through leadership, advocacy, collaboration, outreach, and education. The society is proud to fund and introduce the fifth edition of *Healthy Beginnings* as a uniquely Canadian handbook based on SOGC clinical practice guidelines to give women the information they need to make healthy choices in pregnancy. Proceeds from the sale of the book will be invested in the SOGC's education programs.

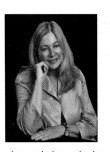

Nan Schuurmans, MD, FRCSC, has been an obstetrician for over 30 years and has delivered more than 5,000 babies. She is currently an Associate Zone Medical Director in Edmonton and a Clinical Professor of Obstetrics and Gynaecology at the University of Alberta.

Throughout her career, she has worked to improve the medical care of women and families and has encouraged women to learn about their own health through knowledge and communication. She led the development of one of Canada's first programs involving home visits for new mothers and babies after early discharge and for women with pregnancy complications previously requiring hospitalization.

Dr. Schuurmans also advanced team care involving nurses, midwives, family doctors, and obstetricians for hard-to-reach and socially disadvantaged women with particular emphasis on indigenous and immigrant populations. She won three REACH awards (Recognizing Excellence and Achievements in Capital Health) for her work in this area in Edmonton. She is a past-president of the SOGC.

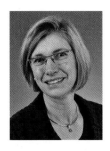

Jennifer Blake, MD, FRCSC, is Chief Executive Officer of the SOGC. During her 30-year career, she has held several clinical, academic, and leadership roles, including Chief of Obstetrics and Gynaecology and Head of Women's Health at the Sunnybrook Health Sciences Centre, Chief of Paediatric Gynaecology at the Hospital for Sick Children in Toronto, and Undergraduate Dean of McMaster University's medical school. She has also served as Professor and Associate Chair at the University of Toronto, as well as Head of Paediatric Gynaecology for the school. She is an Adjunct Professor at the University of Ottawa. In 2011, Dr. Blake was identified as one of the top 25 women of influence in Canada.

CHAPTER ONE

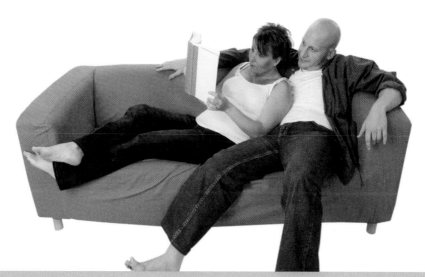

Planning a healthy pregnancy

YOUR MENSTRUAL CYCLE

Almost every woman's menstrual cycle (the time from the first day of the menstrual period to the first day of the next period) varies slightly from month to month. The average length is 28 days, but it can range from 21 to 36 days and often changes with age.

Hormones produced by your body control the changes that occur throughout your cycle. Hormones cause an egg to mature in the ovary and control when the mature egg will be released into your body (ovulation). Ovulation starts about 14 days before your next period.

Preconception—*the time before the baby is conceived—and* **early pregnancy**—*the first 3 months after conception—are important times to make healthy choices that will give you and your baby a healthy beginning.*

Most women understand how important it is to take good care of themselves and their unborn child once they are pregnant. What you may not realize is that the healthy choices you and your partner make before conception will also make a difference to you and your unborn child. You should be aware that you can make the biggest difference to the health of the fetus in the early weeks of pregnancy—before you have missed your period and before you know that you are pregnant.

If you are sexually active, there is always a chance that you might get pregnant. About half of all pregnancies are not planned. If you are planning a pregnancy, understanding your body can help you become pregnant, as well as help you plan a healthy pregnancy.

In this chapter, we'll look at the following:

- *How your body changes in the early stages of pregnancy*
- *What you can do to improve your chances of having a healthy pregnancy and a healthy baby—even before conception takes place*
- *How to avoid hazards that may harm you and your baby*

It all begins with an egg

At a certain time during a woman's monthly menstrual cycle, an egg is released from an ovary. This is called **ovulation.** The egg then begins to move down the fallopian tube toward the uterus. If a sperm enters the egg, **fertilization** takes place. The fertilized egg becomes an **embryo,** which begins to grow immediately.

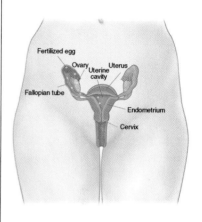

The embryo continues to move down the fallopian tube to the uterus. This takes about 7 days. When it reaches the uterus, the embryo attaches to the thickened lining of the uterus (the endometrium). This is called **implantation**.

For the first 8 weeks, the fertilized egg is called an **embryo**. After 8 weeks, and until birth, the embryo is called a **fetus**.

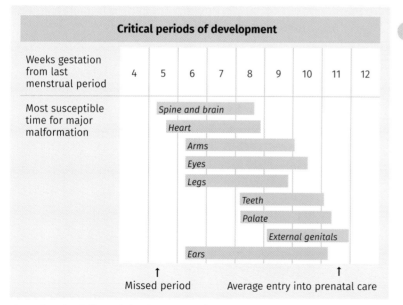

Critical periods of development								
Weeks gestation from last menstrual period	4	5	6	7	8	9	10	11	12
Most susceptible time for major malformation	Spine and brain — Heart — Arms — Eyes — Legs — Teeth — Palate — External genitals — Ears							

↑ Missed period   ↑ Average entry into prenatal care

Source: Reproduced with permission of the March of Dimes.

WHY IS BEING HEALTHY BEFORE CONCEPTION IMPORTANT?

The time when a fetus is most likely to be harmed during pregnancy is also the time when many women may not know they are pregnant. This is between 17 and 56 days after conception, or 4 to 10 weeks from your last menstrual period. At this time, alcohol, certain infections, or a lack of vital nutrients, particularly folic acid, for example, can cause serious harm to the fetus.

How your body supports new life

During the 9 months you are pregnant, your body will provide your baby with everything needed to live and grow. The uterus protects the fetus in a sac filled with liquid (amniotic fluid). All the nutrients and oxygen the fetus needs will come from the **placenta,** which begins to develop where the embryo is implanted in your uterus. The placenta is made up of blood vessels and tissue. It is firmly attached to the lining of your uterus and is essential throughout your pregnancy.

The **umbilical cord** is the lifeline that links your baby to the placenta and to you. The placenta is like a trading post for the blood supply passing between you and your baby. It's where nutrients, oxygen, and protective antibodies travel from your blood to your baby's blood. On the return trip, fetal waste travels from your baby's blood into your bloodstream and is removed by your organs.

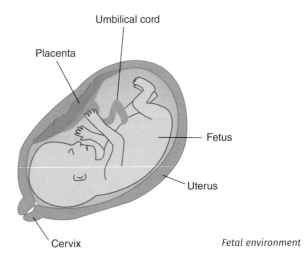

Umbilical cord

Placenta

Fetus

Uterus

Cervix

Fetal environment

The placenta also produces hormones, such as estrogen and progesterone. These hormones cause many of the changes that occur in your body during pregnancy. One of the most important hormones, which only the placenta can produce, is called human chorionic gonadotrophin (HCG). When you take a pregnancy test, the test tells you whether or not this hormone is in your urine or blood. If it is, you are pregnant!

Visit your health care provider before you get pregnant

If you are planning a pregnancy, make an appointment for a check-up with your health care provider. The purpose of this visit

TIPS FOR WHEN YOU VISIT YOUR HEALTH CARE PROVIDER

Every time you see your health care provider, consult these tips. They will help you be organized and feel comfortable.

- *BEFORE your appointment, write down your questions and any details you want to share. Ask your partner, a family member, or a friend to come with you. Two sets of ears are always better than one.*

- *DURING your appointment, ask questions, and ask for a clear answer if you do not really understand what was said. Write things down and keep your notes. Or ask the person accompanying you to take notes for you.*

- *BEFORE you leave your appointment, check that you have asked all the questions on your list and that you understand what your health care provider told you. Make sure you know what will happen next, when your next appointment will be, and if there are any tests planned. Make sure you know whom to contact if you have any problems or questions.*

Source: Adapted from the UK National Health Service's leaflet "Questions to ask."

I DON'T HAVE TO MENTION THAT, DO I?

When you are talking about your health, and your baby's health, be direct and fully honest about your history and lifestyle.

Your health care team needs to see the whole picture to help you plan for a healthy pregnancy and birth.

DO YOU HAVE A HEALTH CARE PROVIDER?

Regular health care is important during pregnancy. If you live in a rural or remote community, you might have limited access to prenatal care. Now is a good time to contact your local health centre, clinic, or nursing station to discuss what is available. Doing so will help you and your future baby get the best care possible.

EARLY SIGNS OF PREGNANCY

- *You missed your period.*

- *You feel more tired than usual.*

- *Your breasts feel tingly or tender.*

- *You need to urinate often.*

- *You feel bloated.*

- *You feel nauseous (morning sickness).*

- *You have unusual bleeding (different from your normal period).*

Any one of these signs, combined with a missed period, could mean you are pregnant (even if you have been using a reliable form of birth control).

is to make sure you are in good health and that your lifestyle will support a healthy baby. Be prepared to give honest answers about your medical history, your family, any medications you take, your diet, your past pregnancies, your sexual history, and the kind of work you do. Your health and your baby's health may depend on this important information. If you are in good health, you probably won't need to see your health care provider again until you suspect you are pregnant.

Learn about pregnancy

As you plan to start or add to your family, it is a good time to learn what to expect during pregnancy and how to prepare for childbirth. This is also a good time to learn about breastfeeding. Women who learn about pregnancy are most likely to have a more positive childbirth experience. Your health care provider and prenatal classes are good sources of information, and women say that what they learned helped them feel more in control throughout their pregnancy and in childbirth. They also felt more fulfilled during the experience.

- Women who take prenatal education say they need less medicine to control pain during labour. This suggests they had less pain or they knew how to cope better with the pain they had.
- Women are more likely to carry their babies to full term when they know about the risk factors that can cause a preterm birth (see page 99).

As you plan, remember that you play an important role in having a healthy pregnancy and a healthy baby. Regular prenatal care and keeping yourself healthy and informed are excellent ways to give your baby a healthy beginning.

WOMEN AGED 35 AND OLDER

Most women aged 35 and older will have a healthy pregnancy and a healthy baby. But some women in this age group are more likely to have certain difficulties when they are pregnant. They may need to take special precautions. If you are in this age group, you should be aware of the following:

- *It may take longer to become pregnant.*

- *You have a higher chance of not being able to get pregnant.*

- *You have a higher chance of having twins or triplets (a multiple birth).*

- *You have a higher chance of having a miscarriage or a baby with a chromosome abnormality.*

- *You have a higher chance of getting diabetes or high blood pressure when you are pregnant.*

- *You have a higher chance of a caesarean birth.*

It is important to remember that most babies are born healthy. The chance of having a baby with a chromosome condition increases with the age of the mother. The age of the father also matters. Semen quality and male fertility decline with advancing age and increase the risk of genetic disorders in offspring. Talk to your health care provider about how you can work together to have the healthiest pregnancy possible. Prenatal tests are available to all women to detect chromosome abnormalities.

Pregnancy and the environment

Most women understand how important it is to take good care of themselves and their unborn child once they are pregnant. What you may not realize is that the healthy choices you and your partner make before conception will also make a difference to you and your unborn child. You should be aware that you can make the biggest difference to the health of the fetus in the early weeks of pregnancy—before you have missed your period and before you know that you are pregnant.

Babies grow in two unique environments. There is the outer environment, where the mother lives. This is a place that we hope includes physical factors such as clean air, pure water, nutritious food, and many family and social supports. The reality is that it is seldom perfect, but this book will provide information and advice on the things that can help make the best environment.

The second environment babies grow in, and the one we usually think of first, is the inner one created in the uterus. This is the dim and watery world where development silently unfolds. Here the mother's health is equally important. This applies to her state of nutrition, the substances she may be using, her state of mental and emotional health, and also the toxins she has been exposed to.

Understanding how our environment from conception affects our health and the health of future generations is a new area of advanced medicine and research. We know that a great many forces from emotional well-being and poverty to chemicals, hormones, and drugs have an effect on the mother, her body, her health, and her growing baby.

In North America, it is estimated that pregnant women can be exposed to at least 43 separate potentially harmful chemicals. They are found in the air, the water, and our food containers, and they make their way into our bodies and from there to our babies. As we learn how toxins and your surroundings can affect your child and your unborn grandchildren, health care providers recommend your pregnancy environment be as healthy and safe as possible.

Things that we can do to ensure healthy beginnings in both the outer and inner pregnancy environments include the following:

- Boost your health by following good nutrition.
- Wash fruits and vegetables well to remove pesticide residues or organic contaminants. Choose fresh or frozen instead of tinned foods.
- Avoid known toxins such as alcohol and tobacco smoke, for example.
- Talk to your health care provider about any toxins you may be exposed to through work.
- Advise your doctor or dentist if you may be pregnant before being exposed to X-rays.
- If you live in a home built before 1950, have the water tested for lead.
- Avoid fish high in mercury.
- Avoid harsh cleaning chemicals and choose vinegar or washing soda, which are environmentally friendly and inexpensive alternatives. Dust and vacuum regularly to remove dust-borne contaminants.
- Your mental and emotional health matters. A strong, supportive family and community are great resources. If you are suffering from depression or living in unsafe circumstances, get help.
- Ask your health care provider about clean air and water. There could be toxic chemicals in the water or the air including mould growing inside your house.
- Ask your elected representatives at the municipal, provincial, territorial, and federal levels to make important changes to protect the air and water around you.

To ensure healthy beginnings for our children, all of us must increase our knowledge and awareness of the world we live in. We must understand its unique risks while doing what we can to protect our own health.

If you are sexually active, there is always a chance that you might get pregnant. About half of all pregnancies are not planned, so it makes sense for all women who may become pregnant to be aware of this health advice.

If you are planning a pregnancy, understanding your body can help you become pregnant as well as help you plan a healthy pregnancy.

Your medical history

Some past or current health problems can affect the outcome of your pregnancy. Women who have serious medical conditions—such as heart disease, diabetes, or high blood pressure—may need additional health care throughout pregnancy by a specialist in that field. Women who are overweight should be tested early in pregnancy for diabetes. If you have epilepsy, talk to your neurologist about your medications before you get pregnant. If you have any medical or mental health condition it is always advisable to meet with your doctor before you become pregnant so that you can be in the best health and on the safest medications. But 50% of all pregnancies are unplanned, so the next best time to speak to your doctor would be as soon as you realize you may be pregnant.

Are you at your healthy weight?

Having a healthy body weight throughout life promotes overall good health and lowers the risk of disease. But everyone is unique. What is a healthy weight for you depends on many factors and varies from woman to woman.

Good health for you and your fetus is not based just on weight. Others factors including good nutrition, regular exercise, good sleeping habits, and a positive attitude will also help you enjoy reduced risks and better health during your pregnancy.

An active life is also important for your health. People need at least two and a half hours of moderate to vigorous intensity aerobic physical activity per week from 18 to 64 years old to enjoy long-term good health. Making changes **before** you get pregnant will help to ensure you have a healthy diet and good exercise habits during pregnancy.

Dietitians of Canada have an online tool to measure body mass index, or BMI. It is a quick screening tool for assessing health based on your height and weight and can be found at www.dietitians.ca/Your-Health/Assess-Yourself/Assess-Your-BMI/BMI-Adult.aspx.

Risks of being overweight: these are some of the things your health care provider will be looking out for

Risks for the mother	Risks for the baby
Infertility	Stillbirth
Miscarriage	Birth defects
Early labour and birth (preterm birth)	Needing to stay in hospital after birth (intensive care)
Diabetes	Grows too big (causing problems during birth)
High blood pressure	
Needing to have a caesarean birth	

MY FAMILY'S MEDICAL HISTORY

List anyone in your close family— such as your parents, brothers, sisters, and children—who has or has had any of these medical conditions:

Diabetes:

A condition that is passed from parent to child (hereditary):

High blood pressure:

A birth defect:

The birth of twins, triplets, or more:

Other problems you think may be serious:

WHAT PRESCRIPTION AND NON-PRESCRIPTION DRUGS, HERBS, AND VITAMINS DO YOU TAKE?

DRUG, HERB, OR VITAMIN
Name:

Amount you take:

How often you take it:

How long you have been taking it:

DRUG, HERB, OR VITAMIN
Name:

Amount you take:

How often you take it:

How long you have been taking it:

DRUG, HERB, OR VITAMIN
Name:

Amount you take:

How often you take it:

How long you have been taking it:

If you are planning to get pregnant and you are concerned that you may be overweight or underweight, you should talk to your health care provider or a registered dietitian about healthy eating.

Medicines and pregnancy

Almost all medicines you take cross through the placenta into a growing baby's body. This includes both prescription and non-prescription medicines. Remember, you share what goes into your body with your baby.

Some medicines are harmful to a growing baby. If you are taking medicines of any kind, it is best to review them with your health care provider before you become pregnant. The chances are good that your health care provider can find a safe alternative for you during pregnancy. If you might become pregnant, it is better to switch to those safer options. It is best to avoid non-prescription drugs, including herbal products, while you are trying to conceive and during pregnancy. Men's exposure to toxic chemicals is also important. Hazardous chemicals at work or recreational drugs can affect a man's fertility. Talk to your health care provider before you use any kind of drug, herb, plant, or home remedy. They will know or find out how safe these products are for pregnant women.

For those medications that we know are harmful, you would have been advised to use effective birth control for as long as you are on that medication. Drugs that are known to cause harm usually do so within the first few weeks of pregnancy—when the baby's major body systems are still forming. If the prescription cannot be changed, your health care provider may advise you to reduce your dosage or to stop using the drug during your pregnancy if it is safe to do so.

If you would like to know more about toxic substances that may harm your baby, talk to the team at the Motherisk Program at the Hospital for Sick Children in Toronto by calling 1–877–439–2744. Or visit their website at www.motherisk.org.

Immunizations and infections

When you are planning your pregnancy, check to see that your immunizations are up-to-date. Infections you can prevent, such as rubella, can harm your unborn baby. It's best to get all your immunizations up-to-date before you become pregnant and then to wait at least 3 months before you conceive. If your immunizations are not up-to-date and you become pregnant, talk to your health care provider.

If your job, lifestyle, or health history makes you more likely to come into contact with illness, your health care provider may recommend that you get vaccines, such as the hepatitis B vaccine.

The Government of Canada has information about immunization for pregnant and breastfeeding women. It is available at www.healthycanadians.gc.ca/healthy-living-vie-saine/ immunization-immunisation/pregnancy-grossesse/index-eng.php.

Immunize Canada has an app that can help you easily record, store, and access vaccine information. Learn more at www.immunize.ca/ en/app.aspx.

Lifestyle and sexual history

You may not feel comfortable talking about your sexual habits, but your health care provider asks these questions to help reduce risks to your baby.

HIV in pregnancy
toll-free helpline
1-888-246-5840

Motherisk's toll-free HIV Healthline offers private advice to Canadian women, their families, and health care providers about the risks of HIV (the human immunodeficiency virus) and HIV treatment in pregnancy. Motherisk also helps HIV specialists and community groups across Canada work together to assess the risks and safety of different HIV treatments.

If you ever have had sex without using a condom—especially if you have had more than one sexual partner—you may have been exposed to a **sexually transmitted infection (STI)** such as genital herpes, genital warts, chlamydia, gonorrhea, syphilis, or the HIV virus.

Some STIs can be cured. Others cannot. Some need to be treated to reduce the risk of infecting the baby at birth.

- Based on your lifestyle and sexual history, certain tests can help you plan your prenatal care.
- HIV testing is offered to all women who are pregnant or are thinking about getting pregnant. The reason? There is a treatment that can greatly reduce the chance that the baby will get HIV from the mother.
- Women who have a disease that comes back again and again— such as genital herpes or genital warts—can still have a normal pregnancy. Sometimes, particularly around the time of the baby's birth, these mothers need special care.

To learn more about STIs, visit www.sexandu.ca.

If you have been pregnant before

Your health care provider will ask you about your past pregnancies and about any problems you may have had during pregnancy, during labour and birth, and after giving birth. Knowing about any previous problems will help your health care provider prevent possible future problems. It's always very important to tell your health care provider as many details as possible about your health so that both of you can plan for any special care you might need.

I have been pregnant before			
	First	Second	Third
Date:			
Where you gave birth (home or name of hospital or birthing centre):			
Hours in labour:			
Type of birth (normal, forceps, C-section):			
Complications or problems:			
Year of birth:			
Baby boy or girl:			
Baby's birth weight:			
Other pregnancies (miscarriages and/or therapeutic abortions):			

Keep track of your monthly cycle

If you are not pregnant, now is a good time to start keeping a record of your menstrual cycle.

A cycle starts on the first day of your period. It ends on the first day of your next period. Then it begins all over again. You can use a calendar to track your cycle. This will help you to predict your next period, know what is normal for you, and figure out when you are most fertile (most likely to conceive). Once you become pregnant, your knowledge of your body's cycles will help your health care provider calculate your **due date**—the day your baby is expected to be born. Your due date and the date of your last menstrual period will also help measure how your baby is growing throughout your pregnancy.

HOW YOUR BODY CHANGES DURING YOUR MENSTRUAL CYCLE

- *A rise in hormone levels changes the lining of the uterus so it is ready to receive the embryo.*
- *The ovary releases an egg (ovulation) about 14 days before the next period begins.*
- *Discharge from your vagina at the time of ovulation becomes more plentiful and clear.*
- *Your body temperature rises for a few days just after ovulation.*
- *You may feel mild cramps in your lower abdomen or bloating near the time of ovulation.*

This chart shows that the first day of this woman's last menstrual period was February 21.

FEBRUARY

S	M	T	W	T	F	S
			1	2	3	4
5	6	7	8	9	10	11
12	13	14	15	16	17	18
19	20	(21)	(22)	(23)	(24)	(25)
26	27	28				

You are most fertile near the time of ovulation. So, if you hope to get pregnant, you and your partner will want to have sexual intercourse around that time. But how can you tell when you are ovulating? The easiest way to tell is to count back 14 days from the day when you predict your next period will start. Most women do not have to do anything else to get pregnant. It just happens naturally.

If you need to be more certain of the best days to try to get pregnant, watch for changes in your body that signal ovulation.

What if I am using the "pill," the "patch," or the "ring"?

If you are using hormonal birth control—such as oral contraceptives (the "pill"), the transdermal patch (the "patch"), or the vaginal ring (the "ring")—you should allow yourself at least one normal menstrual cycle before you try to become pregnant. This will enable your body to have one natural menstrual cycle before becoming pregnant. To protect yourself from pregnancy during this period, use a condom. If you become pregnant while taking hormonal birth control, stop immediately. But don't worry, there are no harmful effects to the baby.

What about other forms of birth control?

If you use an injectable contraceptive (the "shot")—a birth control method that is injected into your body—it may take 6 to 9 months after your last injection before you can become pregnant. You may still safely become pregnant during those months.

If you use spermicidal foams, jellies, condoms, or a diaphragm, you do not have to wait a full cycle before trying to become pregnant. You can start immediately.

If you are using an intrauterine device (IUD) for birth control, you should have it removed before you try to get pregnant. It is not necessary to wait a full cycle after the IUD is removed before you try to get pregnant. If you have an IUD in place and you suspect you may be pregnant, visit your health care provider for a pregnancy test. If you do get pregnant with an IUD in place, talk to your health care provider right away to make sure that you do not have an ectopic (tubal) pregnancy and, if possible, to have the IUD removed. Although it is possible to carry a pregnancy safely with an IUD in place, the IUD can lead to complications such as miscarriage, infection, or preterm birth.

Let's talk about nutrition

Eating well before you become pregnant will help prepare your body to meet the nutritional needs of your developing baby. Follow Eating Well with Canada's Food Guide (see pages 20 and 21) before and during your pregnancy.

- It promotes a wide variety of healthy foods you should eat every day.
- It provides tips and advice for women at all ages and stages of life—such as women who are pregnant, breastfeeding, or are of childbearing age.

By setting good eating habits now, you are likely to find it easier to keep eating well throughout your pregnancy. For most healthy women, following the guide will ensure that you get enough of the vitamins, minerals, and other nutrients you need for a healthy pregnancy. In addition to eating a healthy, balanced diet, pregnant women should also eat often. It's important for pregnant women to avoid long periods without eating (more than 12 hours). The best approach is for pregnant women to eat three meals and three small snacks spread throughout each day. It is also important that women of reproductive age take a multivitamin that contains 0.4 mg of folic acid every day, especially during the 2 to 3 months before they become pregnant. During pregnancy, women need more iron and should take a daily multivitamin that contains 0.4 mg of folic acid and 16–20 mg of iron.

If you have special nutritional needs (see the list in the sidebar on this page and on page 19), talk to your health care provider, who may suggest that you get help from a registered dietitian.

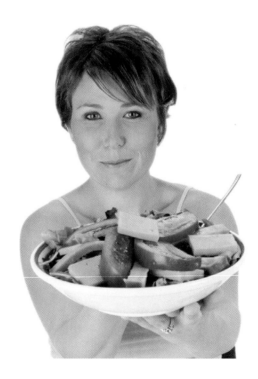

Different people need different amounts of food

The number of servings (from the four food groups) that you need each day is different from other people, depending on your age and whether you are a man or woman. The recommended number of Food Guide servings is an average amount that people should try to eat each day. Women need more calories during the second and third trimesters of pregnancy and when breastfeeding. For most women, this means eating an extra two or three Food Guide servings from any of the food groups each day in addition to their recommended number of Food Guide servings per day. For most women, no additional servings are needed in the first trimester.

How can you get these extra Food Guide servings? Have a snack or add them to your usual meals. For instance, have an extra snack made up of two Food Guide servings or have one extra Food Guide serving of vegetable or fruit at breakfast and one extra Food Guide serving of milk and alternatives at supper.

Canada's Food Guide is available in these languages: Arabic, Chinese, English, Farsi (Persian), French, Korean, Punjabi, Russian, Spanish, Tagalog, Tamil, and Urdu. There is also a Food Guide for First Nations, Inuit, and Métis (see page 21).

NUTRITION QUIZ (CONTINUED)

☐ *I have a serious illness that affects what I can eat.*

☐ *I am under a lot of stress and it affects my food intake.*

☐ *I suffer from serious vomiting problems.*

☐ *I do not have enough money to buy the food I need.*

☐ *I have high cholesterol.*

☐ *I am often constipated (cannot have a bowel movement).*

☐ *I do not eat fish.*

If you checked off any of these boxes, then you have special nutritional needs that you should discuss with your health care provider.

MAKING HEALTHY FOOD CHOICES

EatRight Ontario includes trusted nutrition information written by registered dietitians. It can help you learn how to read and use the nutrition label and also includes a menu planner developed for women who are pregnant. Visit the website at www.eatrightontario.ca.

Eating Well with Canada's Food Guide
Recommended Number of Food Guide Servings per Day—Females ages 19-50

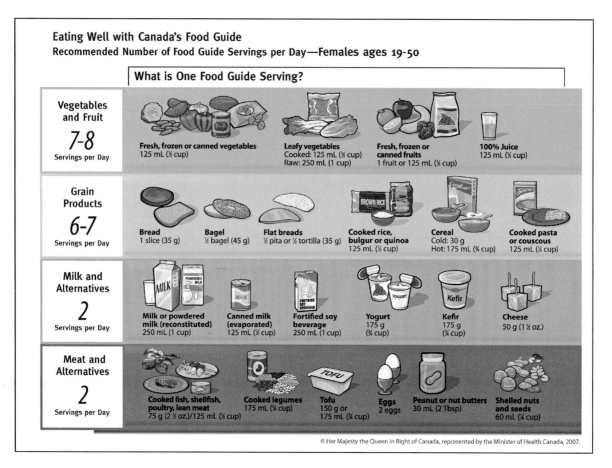

What is One Food Guide Serving?

Vegetables and Fruit
7-8
Servings per Day

- **Fresh, frozen or canned vegetables** 125 mL (½ cup)
- **Leafy vegetables** Cooked: 125 mL (½ cup) Raw: 250 mL (1 cup)
- **Fresh, frozen or canned fruits** 1 fruit or 125 mL (½ cup)
- **100% Juice** 125 mL (½ cup)

Grain Products
6-7
Servings per Day

- **Bread** 1 slice (35 g)
- **Bagel** ½ bagel (45 g)
- **Flat breads** ½ pita or ½ tortilla (35 g)
- **Cooked rice, bulgur or quinoa** 125 mL (½ cup)
- **Cereal** Cold: 30 g Hot: 175 mL (¾ cup)
- **Cooked pasta or couscous** 125 mL (½ cup)

Milk and Alternatives
2
Servings per Day

- **Milk or powdered milk (reconstituted)** 250 mL (1 cup)
- **Canned milk (evaporated)** 125 mL (½ cup)
- **Fortified soy beverage** 250 mL (1 cup)
- **Yogurt** 175 g (¾ cup)
- **Kefir** 175 g (¾ cup)
- **Cheese** 50 g (1 ½ oz.)

Meat and Alternatives
2
Servings per Day

- **Cooked fish, shellfish, poultry, lean meat** 75 g (2 ½ oz.)/125 mL (½ cup)
- **Cooked legumes** 175 mL (¾ cup)
- **Tofu** 150 g or 175 mL (¾ cup)
- **Eggs** 2 eggs
- **Peanut or nut butters** 30 mL (2 Tbsp)
- **Shelled nuts and seeds** 60 mL (¼ cup)

© Her Majesty the Queen in Right of Canada, represented by the Minister of Health Canada, 2007.

Source: Eating Well With Canada's Food Guide (2007), Health Canada. Reproduced with the permission of the Minister of Public Works and Government Services Canada, 2011. www.hc-sc.gc.ca/fn-an/food-guide-aliment/index-eng.php

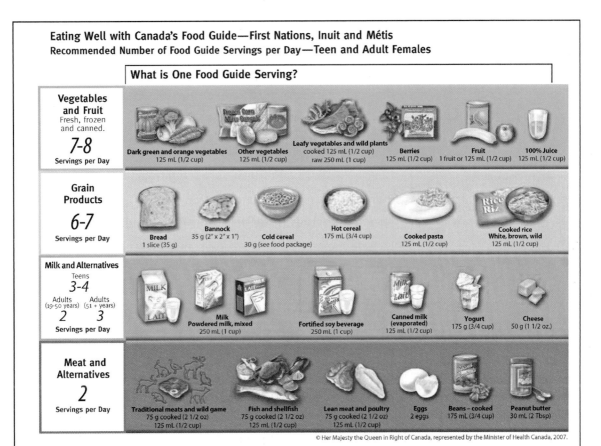

Eating Well with Canada's Food Guide—First Nations, Inuit and Métis
Recommended Number of Food Guide Servings per Day—Teen and Adult Females

What is One Food Guide Serving?

Vegetables and Fruit
Fresh, frozen and canned.
7-8
Servings per Day

- Dark green and orange vegetables 125 mL (1/2 cup)
- Other vegetables 125 mL (1/2 cup)
- Leafy vegetables and wild plants cooked 125 mL (1/2 cup) raw 250 mL (1 cup)
- Berries 125 mL (1/2 cup)
- Fruit 1 fruit or 125 mL (1/2 cup)
- 100% Juice 125 mL (1/2 cup)

Grain Products
6-7
Servings per Day

- Bread 1 slice (35 g)
- Bannock 35 g (2" x 2" x 1")
- Cold cereal 30 g (see food package)
- Hot cereal 175 mL (3/4 cup)
- Cooked pasta 125 mL (1/2 cup)
- Cooked rice White, brown, wild 125 mL (1/2 cup)

Milk and Alternatives
Teens
3-4
Adults (19-50 years) **2**   Adults (51 + years) **3**
Servings per Day

- Milk Powdered milk, mixed 250 mL (1 cup)
- Fortified soy beverage 250 mL (1 cup)
- Canned milk (evaporated) 125 mL (1/2 cup)
- Yogurt 175 g (3/4 cup)
- Cheese 50 g (1 1/2 oz.)

Meat and Alternatives
2
Servings per Day

- Traditional meats and wild game 75 g cooked (2 1/2 oz) 125 mL (1/2 cup)
- Fish and shellfish 75 g cooked (2 1/2 oz) 125 mL (1/2 cup)
- Lean meat and poultry 75 g cooked (2 1/2 oz) 125 mL (1/2 cup)
- Eggs 2 eggs
- Beans – cooked 175 mL (3/4 cup)
- Peanut butter 30 mL (2 Tbsp)

© Her Majesty the Queen in Right of Canada, represented by the Minister of Health Canada, 2007.

Source: Eating Well With Canada's Food Guide—First Nations, Inuit and Métis (2007), Health Canada. Reproduced with the permission of the Minister of Public Works and Government Services Canada, 2011. www.hc-sc.gc.ca/fn-an/food-guide-aliment/fnim-pnim/index-eng.php

Women planning a pregnancy should take a daily multivitamin containing 0.4 mg of folic acid. Pregnant women should take a multivitamin containing 0.4 mg of folic acid and 16–20 mg of iron.

IF IT COSTS TOO MUCH TO EAT WELL

Some women are not always able to buy the food they need to have a healthy pregnancy and baby. Talk to your health care provider or contact your local public health unit for information about food programs in your community.

The Government of Canada provides funding to community groups to support the food needs of pregnant women. A program in your community may be able to provide you with the support you need. To learn more about the Canada Prenatal Nutrition Program, visit the Public Health Agency of Canada's website at www.phac-aspc.gc.ca/hp-ps/dca-dea/prog-ini/cpnp-pcnp/index-eng.php.

Guidelines from Health Canada

Vegetables and fruit

Eat at least one dark green (such as broccoli or spinach) and one orange (such as carrots or sweet potatoes) vegetable each day.

Choose vegetables and fruit prepared with little or no added fat, sugar, or salt. Enjoy vegetables steamed, baked, or stir-fried instead of deep-fried.

Have vegetables and fruits more often than juice.

Grain products

Ensure that at least half your daily grain products are whole grain.

Include bread, pasta, rice, cereal, and other grains, such as barley, oats, and quinoa.

Enjoy whole-grain breads, oatmeal, or whole-wheat pasta.

Choose grain products that are low in fat, sugar, and salt. Compare products and make wise choices by reading the Nutrition Facts label.

Milk and alternatives

Have 500 ml (2 cups) of milk every day.

Drink fortified non-dairy alternative beverages if you do not drink milk.

Compare the Nutrition Facts label on non-dairy alternative beverages, yogurts, or cheeses to help make healthy choices.

Meat and alternatives

Have meat and alternatives such as beans, lentils, and tofu often.

Select lean meat and alternatives prepared with little or no added fat or salt.

Trim the visible fat from meats and remove the skin from poultry. Use cooking methods such as roasting, baking, or poaching, which require little or no added fat.

Include at least two Food Guide servings of low-mercury fish each week (see list of fish on pages 24 and 25).

Unsaturated fat

For good health, include a small amount (30–45 ml/2–3 tbsp) of unsaturated fat each day. This amount includes oil used for cooking, salad dressings, margarine, and mayonnaise. Unsaturated vegetable oils include canola, corn, flaxseed, olive, peanut, soybean, and sunflower.

Foods to limit or avoid during pregnancy

Foods that may contain bacteria

Foods that contain bacteria and parasites are very risky for pregnant women and their unborn children. For example, listeriosis is a rare but serious disease. It can cause miscarriage, stillbirth, illness in the mother, and severe illness in the newborn.

To prevent infections from food, pregnant women should avoid the following:

- Raw seafood, such as sushi, raw oysters, clams, and mussels (stick with sushi made only with vegetables or cooked fish to be safe)
- Refrigerated smoked seafood
- Undercooked meat, poultry, and seafood (for example, hot dogs straight from the package, without further heating; non-dried deli meats, such as bologna, roast beef, and turkey breast; refrigerated pâté; meat spreads; and refrigerated smoked seafood and fish)

COMMON THINGS TO AVOID OR LIMIT WHEN YOU ARE PREGNANT

Alcohol
- *Do not drink any kind of alcohol in any amount.*

Caffeine
- *Limit yourself to 300 mg of caffeine per day. For reference, this is the amount found in 2 to 3 cups of coffee or 6 cups of black tea. Carbonated beverages can contain high levels of caffeine so it is best to check the labels. Chocolate also contains small amounts of caffeine.*
- *Avoid energy drinks.*

Herbs and herbal teas
- *Some teas are safe if you drink moderately (2 or 3 cups a day). Good choices are citrus peel, ginger, lemon, orange peel, echinacea, peppermint, rosemary, red raspberry leaf, and rose hip.*
- *Herbal supplements are not recommended.*
- *Some herbs are not safe to take during pregnancy. It is best to check any herbal preparation for safety in pregnancy.*

Artificial sweeteners
- *Products containing artificial sweeteners should not be used in place of nutrient-rich foods. If you do use them, please do so in moderation.*

- All foods made with raw or lightly cooked eggs (for example, homemade Caesar vinaigrette, some salad dressings, cookie dough, cake batter, sauces, and drinks such as homemade eggnog)
- Raw or unpasteurized milk products
- Unpasteurized and pasteurized soft cheeses, such as Brie and Camembert
- Unpasteurized and pasteurized semi-soft cheeses, such as Havarti
- All unpasteurized and pasteurized blue-veined cheeses
- Unpasteurized juices, such as unpasteurized apple cider
- Raw sprouts, especially alfalfa sprouts

Do not store fresh or cooked meat or poultry in the refrigerator for longer than 2 or 3 days. Keep uncooked meats separate from other foods. Wash hands, cooking utensils, and cooking surfaces well after handling uncooked meat. Wash raw vegetables (especially pre-cut and ready-to-eat vegetables) thoroughly before eating. Wash reusable shopping bags often.

Important facts about fish

Fish is an especially important food in pregnancy because it is a good source of protein and omega-3 fatty acids. Regular consumption of fish during pregnancy plays a role in normal fetal brain and eye development. Canada's Food Guide recommends eating at least 150 grams (two Food Guide servings) of fish each week.

Some types of fish have higher levels of beneficial fatty acids than others. Fish and shellfish that contain higher levels of these fatty acids and are also low in mercury include anchovy, capelin, char, hake, herring, Atlantic mackerel, mullet, pollock (Boston bluefish), salmon, smelt, rainbow trout, lake whitefish, haddock, cod, and sardines.

Fish may contain bacteria that are harmful in pregnancy. Freezing raw fish for 4 days will kill parasites but may not kill all disease-causing microorganisms, so cooked fish is the safest choice in pregnancy.

Some types of fish contain higher levels of mercury than others. Mercury may hinder brain development in your baby. Limit the kinds of fish that have high mercury content to no more than 150 grams or two Food Guide servings per month.

Women who are trying to get pregnant or who are pregnant or breastfeeding should limit consumption to 150 grams per month of the following fish: fresh or frozen tuna, shark, swordfish, marlin, orange roughy, and escolar.

Pregnant women should also limit consumption of canned Albacore "white" tuna to 300 grams a week. Canned Albacore tuna is also often called canned white tuna. It is not the same as canned light tuna. Canned light tuna contains other species of tuna such as skipjack, yellowfin, and tongol, which have less mercury.

To learn more about mercury in fish in Canada, visit www.hc-sc .gc.ca/fn-an/securit/chem-chim/environ/mercur/cons-adv-etud-eng.php.

The levels of mercury in fresh water fish (locally fished) can vary. To find out about any fish advisories from provincial and territorial authorities before eating a particular fish, see   www.ec.gc.ca/mercure-mercury/default.asp?lang=En&n=DCBE5083–1.

For more details on foods to avoid during pregnancy, see the Government of Canada's Health and Safety website at www.healthycanadians.gc.ca.

Other important nutrients

Omega-3 fatty acids

These types of fats are considered healthy (your body needs them and so does your baby) and essential because your body cannot make them by itself. You must get omega-3 fatty acids through

Fish is an excellent source of protein and omega-3 fatty acids. Both are very important for your baby's growth and development. Check this section (pages 24 and 25) for a list of fish to choose more often.

- *Salmon and other cold-water fish such as char, herring, mackerel, sardines, and trout*

- *Omega-3 fortified eggs*

- *Walnut oil*

- *Flax oil*

- *Vegetable oils such as olive, canola, soybean, and soft (non-hydrogenated) margarine*

the food you eat (refer to the list in the sidebar "Food sources of omega-3 fatty acids"). Omega-3 fatty acids have been linked to health benefits for your heart, your joints, and your mental health. They have also been linked to better blood flow to the placenta and the growing baby, and they may help to prevent preterm labour. In a growing baby, these fats support development of the brain and nervous system. They also improve the baby's vision and skin. The best source of omega-3 fatty acids is fish. Health Canada recommends that pregnant women should consume at least two servings (75 g each) of fish each week.

Minerals and vitamins

Do I need to take special vitamins?

Women planning a pregnancy should take a daily multivitamin containing folic acid. Pregnant women need a multivitamin containing folic acid and iron. **Folic acid** will help your baby grow and will help prevent certain birth defects. Following Canada's Food Guide and taking a multivitamin a day will help you meet your nutrient needs during pregnancy.

What about the dangers of too much of a vitamin?

Taking more than the recommended dose of vitamins can be harmful. For example, too much vitamin A (more than 10,000 IU/3,000 µg RAE [retinol activity equivalents] per day) is linked to birth defects. Make sure you do not take more than one tablet per day of your multivitamin. Read the label on any vitamins you buy. If you have doubts about a vitamin, ask your health care provider before you take it. Your health care provider may suggest advice from a registered dietitian.

Calcium and vitamin D

Women who are pregnant or breastfeeding need calcium and vitamin D to maintain bone strength. Pregnant women need both to build the baby's bones. The recommended daily intake for calcium is 1,000 μg/day. For vitamin D, it is 15 μg/day (600 IU). Extra calcium is better absorbed when you take it between meals and at different times.

Milk and alternatives such as cheese and yogurt are at the top of the list of good sources of calcium, and the kind of calcium they contain is easily absorbed by the body. Milk and fortified soy beverages are enriched with vitamin D, which also helps you absorb calcium. See the "Dietary sources of calcium" list for other good sources of calcium.

Women may be at risk of poor vitamin D status, particularly if they do not have 2 cups of milk or fortified soy beverages every day. If you think you may not be getting enough calcium or vitamin D, talk to your health care provider or a registered dietitian about vitamin supplements.

Dietary sources of calcium

	Serving size		Calcium (mg)
VEGETABLES AND FRUITS			
Vegetables			
Collards, frozen, cooked	125 ml	(1/2 cup)	189
Spinach, frozen, cooked	125 ml	(1/2 cup)	154
Fruit			
Orange juice, fortified with calcium	125 ml	(1/2 cup)	155
MILK AND ALTERNATIVES			
Buttermilk	250 ml	(1 cup)	370
Almond milk, fortified with calcium	250 ml	(1 cup)	Up to 450
Soy beverage, fortified with calcium	250 ml	(1 cup)	321 to 324
3.25% homo, 2%, 1%, skim, chocolate milk	250 ml	(1 cup)	291 to 322
Dry powdered milk	24 g (4 tbsp) to make 250 ml of milk		302
CHEESE			
Gruyere, Swiss, goat, low-fat cheddar, mozzarella	50 g	(1½ oz)	396 to 506
Processed cheese slices (Swiss, cheddar, low-fat Swiss)	50 g	(1½ oz)	276 to 386
Cheddar, Colby, Edam, Gouda, mozzarella	50 g	(1½ oz)	252 to 366
Ricotta cheese	125 ml	(1/2 cup)	269 to 356
Cottage cheese	250 ml	(1 cup)	146 to 217
MISCELLANEOUS			
Yogurt, plain	175 g	(3/4 cup)	292 to 332
Yogurt, fruit bottom	175 g	(3/4 cup)	221 to 291
Yogurt, soy	175 g	(3/4 cup)	206
Yogurt beverage	200 ml		190
Kefir	175 g	(3/4 cup)	187
FISH			
Sardines, Atlantic, canned in oil, with bones	75 g	(2½ oz)	286
Salmon (pink/humpback, red/sockeye), canned, with bones	75 g	(2½ oz)	179 to 208
Mackerel, canned	75 g	(2½ oz)	181
Sardines, Pacific, canned in tomato sauce, with bones	75 g	(2½ oz)	180
Anchovies, canned	75 g	(2½ oz)	174
MEAT ALTERNATIVES			
Tofu, prepared with calcium sulfate	150 g	(3/4 cup)	234 to 347
OTHER			
Goat's milk or rice beverage, fortified with calcium	250 ml	(1 cup)	319 to 345
Blackstrap molasses	15 ml	(1 tbsp)	179

Source: Adapted from Dietitians of Canada. Food Sources of Calcium.

Folic acid

Folic acid is a vitamin that helps prevent neural tube defects (NTDs). It may also prevent other birth defects. The risk of having a baby with NTDs (which affect the baby's brain and spinal cord) is lower if women take a daily vitamin that contains folic acid before they become pregnant and during the early weeks of pregnancy. Women of reproductive age should take a daily multivitamin that contains 0.4 mg of folic acid, especially during the 2 to 3 months before they become pregnant, during pregnancy and breastfeeding.

NTDs occur when a baby's spinal cord, skull, or brain does not develop normally between the third and the fourth week of pregnancy. During this time, many women do not even know they are pregnant.

Women at higher risk (see "Folic acid quiz") may benefit from taking more folic acid. You should discuss this with your health care provider.

Food sources of folic acid

(Based on usual serving size)

EXCELLENT SOURCES OF FOLIC ACID
55 µG (MCG) OR MORE

Cooked beans (fava, kidney, pinto, roman, soy, and white), chickpeas, lentils
Cooked spinach, asparagus
Romaine lettuce
Orange juice, canned pineapple juice
Sunflower seeds

GOOD SOURCES OF FOLIC ACID
33 µG (MCG) OR MORE

Cooked lima beans, corn, broccoli, green peas, Brussels sprouts, beets
Bean sprouts
Oranges
Honeydew melon
Raspberries, blackberries
Avocado
Wheat germ

OTHER SOURCES OF FOLIC ACID
11 µG (MCG) OR MORE

Cooked carrots, beet greens, sweet potato, snow peas, summer and winter squash, rutabaga, cabbage, green beans
Cashews, walnuts
Eggs
Strawberries, banana, grapefruit, cantaloupe
Whole-wheat or white bread
Pork, kidney
Breakfast cereals
Milk, all types

FOLIC ACID QUIZ

Do you need extra folic acid before and during pregnancy? Check off any statements in the following list that are true for you.

☐ *I have epilepsy.*

☐ *I have anemia.*

☐ *I have diabetes that requires me to take insulin.*

☐ *I or my partner had a previous pregnancy in which the baby had a birth defect (see sidebar on page 30).*

☐ *Either I have—or my partner has—a close relative who was born with a birth defect (see sidebar on page 30).*

☐ *I use alcohol or recreational drugs (see pages 36 to 38).*

☐ *I do not eat healthy foods each day (see page 17).*

☐ *My BMI is 30 or more (see page 11).*

☐ *I smoke.*

If you are planning a pregnancy and you checked any of the preceding boxes, you should talk to your health care provider about the right amount of folic acid to take.

Folic acid and other vitamins are very important to your growing baby's health and development (see "Do I need to take special vitamins?" on page 26). Talk to your health care provider or community health nurse if you cannot find or buy the vitamins you need.

In Canada, folic acid is added to all white flour, enriched pasta, and cornmeal products. Women who consume a gluten-free diet may have a lower folic acid intake.

Anemia and iron

Hemoglobin is a substance found in the blood. It carries oxygen from your lungs to other parts of your body and to your growing baby. You need more iron during pregnancy to support increases in your own blood volume and the growth of your baby. Anemia means that you have lower levels of hemoglobin in your blood. During pregnancy, a woman may develop anemia because she has low levels of iron in her body. Low iron levels contribute to fatigue, low infant birth weight, preterm birth, and other complications for both you and your baby.

If you are taking a multivitamin with the recommended 16–20 mg of iron, it is better absorbed when you take it between meals. Your health care provider can help you determine the vitamins that are right for you.

The sidebar "Dietary sources of iron" on page 31 will help guide you to iron-rich foods. Our bodies absorb iron from animal sources better than iron from non-animal sources. Vitamin C helps your body absorb iron. This means if you have a glass of orange juice (vitamin C) with your boiled egg (iron), you will be helping your body absorb the iron better.

Your health care provider may also perform a blood test to find out if your hemoglobin level is normal (between 110 and 112 g/L).

Iodine

Iodine is a mineral found in very small quantities in the body. It is used to make thyroid hormone. Thyroid hormone is important for muscles, bone development, and helps with nutrient absorption. Your body needs extra iodine during pregnancy. The main source of iodine in the diet is iodized table salt. Because people are consuming less table salt or are choosing non-iodized salt such as sea salt, low iodine levels are becoming more common. You can ensure you are getting enough iodine by taking a daily prenatal multivitamin during pregnancy. Be sure your table salt is iodized.

Dietary sources of iron

(Milligrams [mg] of iron found in each 100-gram portion)

EXCELLENT SOURCES OF IRON

Liver (Even though this is an excellent source, you should eat no more than 75 grams [2.5 oz] of liver once every 2 weeks if you are pregnant because of the high levels of vitamin A in liver. Too much vitamin A can cause birth defects in pregnancy.)

GOOD SOURCES OF IRON

Beef (3.1–3.9 mg), veal (3.2–3.6 mg), shrimp (2.1–3.4 mg)

SOURCES OF IRON

Blackstrap molasses (3.6 mg of iron in 15 ml [1 tbsp] serving)
Lamb (2.0 mg), dark-meat poultry (1.3 mg), pork (1.1 mg)

OTHER SOURCES OF IRON

Egg yolk, legumes, tofu
Dark green vegetables (spinach, broccoli, peas)
Dried fruit
Breakfast cereals enriched with iron
Pumpkin seeds

Nutrition tracking

Use this chart to keep track of your eating habits for one week. Then compare your habits with the recommendations in *Eating Well with Canada's Food Guide.* Use this as a guide to eating during your pregnancy. Mark an x for each serving you have eaten during the day.

	Vegetables & Fruit 7–8 servings	Grain Products 6–7 servings	Milk & Alternatives 2 servings	Meat & Alternatives 2 servings	Additional Servings 2–3 servings (recommended for the second and third trimesters)
Day 1					
Day 2					
Day 3					
Day 4					
Day 5					
Day 6					
Day 7					

Vegetarian diets

A carefully planned vegetarian diet is healthy during pregnancy and when breastfeeding. Extra attention to protein is needed. Strict vegetarians (vegans) should also pay careful attention to their need for zinc, iron, vitamin B12, and omega-3 fatty acids.

Exercise

Women who are physically fit before pregnancy have fewer aches and pains and more energy during their pregnancy. You do not need to be an athlete. Just being active on a regular basis (walking, swimming, or doing yoga, etc.) makes a difference to being a healthy weight and your general well-being.

If you have been active for at least 6 months, ask about whether you can continue your sports or workouts safely. As you move further into your pregnancy and your body naturally changes, you may feel mild aches and pains because of looser joints and shifting of your body weight. It may be a good idea to revise your exercise program every trimester to reduce the risk of falling. You should also ask your health care provider about limiting high-impact activities. Certain high-risk activities such as scuba diving are not recommended.

If you have not been active and would like to begin an activity program, "start low and go slow." Exercise is good for you and your baby and, for almost all pregnant women, it is highly recommended. Try regular brisk walking, swimming, strength training for pregnant women, or other activities that will strengthen your heart and lungs and tone your muscles. If you are not physically active when you become pregnant, wait until the second trimester to start your program. You can read more about exercise during pregnancy in Chapter Two.

WHY SHOULD YOU QUIT SMOKING?

- *My baby will get more oxygen from me.*

- *My baby will be less likely to have breathing problems after she is born.*

- *My baby will be more likely to be a normal weight when he is born.*

- *My baby will be less likely to be born early.*

- *My baby will be more likely to grow and develop normally.*

- *I will breathe better and have more energy.*

- *I will save money.*

- *I will feel good about myself for making a healthy decision for me and my baby.*

Workplace

Women planning a pregnancy should follow all safety rules if they must work with chemicals, solvents, fumes, or radiation. If you are already pregnant, your health care provider may advise you to avoid any contact with some of these workplace hazards. See the Motherisk website (www.motherisk.org) for more details about exposure risks at work and at home during pregnancy.

Shift work, doing very demanding physical work, working long hours, and having to commute a long distance can increase the risk of miscarriage or having a small or preterm baby. You can read more about how we define very demanding physical (strenuous) work during pregnancy in Chapter Three.

Employers have a duty to accommodate for pregnancy-related conditions and circumstances including breastfeeding. Visit the Canadian Human Rights Commission website to get more information www.chrc-ccdp.gc.ca/eng/content/policy-and-best-practices-page-1.

Smoking

The risks of smoking during pregnancy are well known. Cigarette smoke contains thousands of compounds including arsenic, formaldehyde, and carbon monoxide. Smoking can also lead to small or preterm babies. There is also a great deal of evidence that second-hand smoke harms infants and children. If you or your partner smokes, an excellent way to prepare for being a parent is to **stop smoking now.** Smoking cessation is the most important step you can take to improving your health, and the health of your baby.

If you are already pregnant and still smoking, there are aids such as nicotine replacement treatments in a patch, an inhaler, or gum that can help with withdrawal symptoms and cigarette cravings while increasing the likelihood of success. These are safe to use during pregnancy but higher doses may be required. Nicotine is metabolized more quickly during pregnancy, making cravings stronger. You and your baby are much safer when you use nicotine replacement treatments than when you are smoking. Talk to your health care provider to learn more. E-cigarettes have not been tested in pregnancy.

Talk to your health care provider to learn about programs and treatments that can help with smoking cessation. If you quit smoking before you reach your 16th week, there is less chance that your baby will be born too early or be too small. Babies born too early and too small (underweight) face some additional health challenges. They are also more likely to have problems sleeping and eating, more likely to get sick, and can have long-term health problems. The best way to proceed, if you are planning to have a baby, is to quit smoking **before** you get pregnant. This way, your baby will enjoy the most health benefits. However, it is important to be aware that there are health benefits to quitting at any time, even after your child is born.

A lot of help is out there to quit smoking. PREGNETS has the most up-to-date information on smoking-cessation practices for pregnant and postpartum women, an anonymous online discussion board, and a personalized plan for quitting or reducing smoking at www.pregnets.org. Another good resource is The Canadian Cancer Society's Smokers' Helpline, which connects you with a quit coach at 1–877–513–5333, or Smokers Helpline Online at www.smokershelpline.ca/how-to-get-help.

I CAN QUIT SMOKING! (CONTINUED)

WHAT ABOUT THE PEOPLE AROUND ME?

- *I will ask others not to smoke around me.*
- *I will go to non-smoking areas when I go out.*

DOUBLE TROUBLE

Quitting smoking is never easy. It can be tougher during pregnancy. Pregnant women process nicotine from cigarettes much faster, which means nicotine cravings can be stronger, making it more difficult to resist smoking. Quitting before getting pregnant would be much easier! A lot of help is available if you are pregnant and still smoking and want to cut down or quit.

(See "Smoking cessation" on p. 247 to find help to get past the cravings and help you quit altogether.)

Alcohol

Alcohol may be part of your lifestyle, and if it is ask yourself if you are able to make some healthy changes on your own or if you will need help. Alcohol or drugs can contribute to the risk of an unplanned pregnancy, and they can affect your health and the health of your baby.

We live in a society that can make those choices feel difficult. Many women, knowing the risks, continue to accept drinks or recreational drugs rather than have friends know that they are pregnant, or they may feel pressure by their friends or partners to continue. There is help available if you are under these pressures.

Because of potential serious health risks to a developing baby, women are advised not to drink any alcohol if they are pregnant or planning to become pregnant.

- There is no known safe amount of alcohol during pregnancy.
- There is no safe kind of alcohol during pregnancy.
- There is no safe time for alcohol use in pregnancy.
- The more alcohol a woman drinks, the greater the risks to her unborn baby.

Alcohol can cause serious brain damage and other health risks for a growing baby. These effects last a lifetime. Babies can have difficulty learning and remembering, slow development, problems getting along with others, and birth defects.

How harmful will a pregnant woman's drinking be? It depends on many factors, such as your own health, complex interactions between you and your developing baby, how much you drink, and when. The safest choice is not to drink at all if you might become pregnant and during pregnancy. Even low to moderate levels of alcohol use in pregnancy can harm the fetus, with life-long consequences.

Alcohol is harmful to my baby

Fetal alcohol spectrum disorder (FASD) is the term used to describe the range of disabilities and diagnoses that result from a mother's drinking alcohol during pregnancy. Those who live with FASD may have mild to very severe problems such as:

- Learning disabilities, particularly in mathematical concepts
- Difficulty understanding the consequences of their actions
- Mental health issues
- Physical disabilities, such as kidney and internal organ problems
- Skeletal abnormalities

There is no cure for FASD. People live with FASD for their entire lives, so early intervention is key to minimizing the disabilities associated with it. People with FASD may need continued support throughout their lives to deal with their difficulties. Visit Health Canada's website to get more information: www.hc-sc.gc.ca/hl-vs/iyh-vsv/diseases-maladies/fasd-etcaf-eng.php.

Cannabis

Cannabis use may affect the baby's development during pregnancy and after the baby is born. Cannabis use during pregnancy is linked with slow growth during pregnancy and low birth weight. While the evidence is mixed, heavier use may result in more harm.

FOR MORE INFORMATION
ABOUT FASD

Canadian Centre on Substance Abuse

1-613-235-4048

www.ccsa.ca

Motherisk Alcohol and Substance Use Helpline

1-877-327-4636

www.motherisk.org

NO, THANKS, MY BABY IS TOO YOUNG TO DRINK!

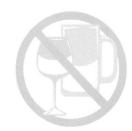

Other drugs

Using drugs at any time during pregnancy may cause damage to your growing baby. Drugs can be harmful to an adult, but they can severely affect the earliest stages of a baby's development and have longer-term harmful effects that carry into early childhood and beyond. It is difficult to identify the effects of each substance on babies because multiple drugs are often used at the same time.

Medical complications can result from using illegal drugs during pregnancy and can lead to early pregnancy loss, a detached placenta, problems with baby's growth, high blood pressure, stillbirth, preterm labour, and hemorrhaging following labour.

A fetus can become dependent on drugs that are transmitted through the bloodstream.

If you are using drugs, seek help before you get pregnant. If you do become pregnant while still using drugs, tell your health care provider. Programs to help with quitting are available.

My pregnancy journal
My health before pregnancy

NUTRITION QUIZ:

I follow Canada's Food Guide.	Yes/No	I am taking folic acid.	Yes/No
I have enough calcium in my diet.	Yes/No	I have sources of vitamin C, vitamin D, magnesium, zinc, and omega-3 fatty acids in my diet.	Yes/No
I get enough iron from my diet.	Yes/No		

If you answer "no" to any of these questions (or are uncertain), review the chapter information and talk to your health care provider.

_____

_____

_____

_____

_____

_____

_____

_____

_____

_____

_____

KEEPING TRACK OF MY PROGRESS

Date:

Blood pressure:

Weight:

THINGS TO DISCUSS WITH MY HEALTH CARE PROVIDER:

☐ *Concerns about my weight.*

☐ *The kind of work that I do.*

☐ *Quitting smoking.*

☐ *Concerns about alcohol or drugs.*

☐ *My medical history.*

☐ *My family history.*

☐ *Exercise.*

☐ *Other concerns:*

My to-do list

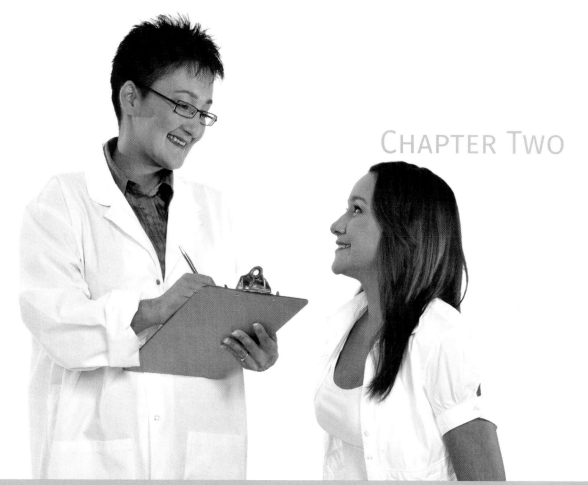

CHAPTER TWO

Off to a great start: the first trimester

WHAT IS A TRIMESTER?

It is common to divide the 9 months of a full pregnancy into three trimesters. Each trimester is about 3 months long. The countdown begins at conception.

- The first trimester starts at conception and goes to the 13th week.

- The second trimester goes from the 13th week to about the 25th or 26th week.

- The third and final trimester lasts from about the 26th week to when the baby is born.

Your first trimester is the time when you and your baby will experience the greatest amount of change. During these 13 weeks, your baby will grow from a single cell to a little living being. At the same time, you will notice changes to your body that may surprise you, especially if this is your first pregnancy.

Finding out you are pregnant can be one of the most exciting moments of your life. This is especially true if you have been planning and hoping to become pregnant for some time. However, the first weeks of your pregnancy may bring some worry along with joy. What is happening to my body? What if something is wrong with my baby? Am I going to feel like this for 9 months?

You will have lots of questions. Feeling some anxiety is perfectly normal. Your health care team is there to help you with answers. They will also recommend some tests for you and your growing baby.

To help you prepare, this chapter will cover a lot of territory. It will explain the tests and the routines of prenatal care that you may be offered by your health care provider as well as the physical changes you may be feeling. You will be able to learn more about common experiences during healthy pregnancy, such as morning sickness, and find answers to common questions, such as if there will be any changes in your sex life. If you and your baby are at risk from any kind of abuse, you will find information on how to get help. And there is information on prenatal classes and exercise—and much much more.

At the end of this chapter you will find a discussion of some topics that you may not want to think about—such as miscarriage. Much of what we will cover in the next pages will help to reduce those risks, but sometimes things simply don't go as we hoped, no matter what you did to make your pregnancy healthy; so we will address what happens if your pregnancy doesn't go well.

By using this handbook and learning as much as you can about what will happen to you and your baby during pregnancy, you will be off to a great start. This book will help you make good choices about your health, nutrition, and lifestyle for you and your baby.

Your changing body

During your first trimester, your body will go through some dramatic changes. By the end of the first 13 weeks, you may not *look* very pregnant, but you will probably *feel* quite different.

At this stage, pregnancy hormones cause almost all the changes in your body. Earlier we discussed *the placenta*. That's the small organ that grows along the inside wall of your uterus to nourish your baby. It also produces hormones to help your body support your baby. This building process is complex and takes a lot of energy. That's one of the reasons you may feel so tired in your early months.

The changes in your body will not be noticed much by other people. You may not even notice that your uterus is slowly growing—from the size of a pear to the size of a cantaloupe. Your milk glands develop and your breasts feel fuller, heavier, and tender. Your heart works harder now because your body is producing extra blood to support the growing placenta and to provide oxygen and nutrients to your baby. You may be more aware of your breathing. Some women feel breathless because of hormone changes. Your menstrual cycle will stop. If you have any bleeding during pregnancy, consult your health care provider right away.

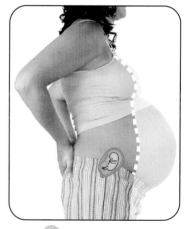

First trimester

Your growing baby

By the end of the first trimester, your 13-week-old fetus will be about 9 cm long (3.5 inches) and weigh about 48 grams (1.7 ounces). Because the baby is so small, it will still have plenty of space to move around freely. Although your baby will be very active, you will not be able to feel the movement until later.

The baby's body will now be fully formed, but it will still need more time to gain weight and to allow its organs to mature. At 13 weeks, the fingers and toes are developed. The bones are mostly soft (cartilage), but they are starting to harden. The head still looks too big compared to the rest of the body. There are signs of 32 tooth buds in the jaw. The heart beats about 140 times per minute.

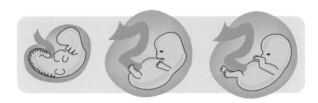

The embryo develops rapidly during the first 8 weeks of pregnancy.

Choosing a health care provider

Prenatal care is delivered by different health care providers, including obstetricians, family doctors, registered midwives, and nurse practitioners.

Routine prenatal care delivered by any of these health care providers is covered by government health plans. It is important that you have a health care provider you trust and feel comfortable with.

Most pregnancies are healthy. This means that the mother is healthy, and the baby is developing normally. When risk factors are present, you may require extra attention and medical care during pregnancy.

Conditions that would increase risk are medical problems of the mother, such as diabetes or high blood pressure, and problems associated with pregnancy itself, such as poor growth of the baby. Concerns related to poverty, lack of emotional support from family and friends, and addictions (cigarettes and alcohol) can also increase risk.

Family physicians, registered midwives, and nurse practitioners are trained to look after normal or low-risk pregnancies and know how to recognize and treat some complications. Obstetricians/ gynaecologists are specialist doctors who regularly look after women with healthy pregnancies but who have extra training in complications of pregnancy and birth and surgical procedures such as caesarean births. Sometimes family doctors, particularly if working in rural areas, may also have the extra training required to do caesarean births.

All of these health care professionals are capable of taking care of women with normal, low-risk pregnancies. Sometimes a referral to an obstetrician for advice or care is necessary, but many times the obstetrician will work with you and your family physician or midwife, as a member of the team.

How often should I expect to visit my health care provider?

Your first visit should be booked as soon as you think you are pregnant. For the rest of the first trimester, you should see your health care provider at least once every 4 weeks. After 30 weeks, the visits are usually increased to once every 2 to 3 weeks. After 36 weeks, you should see your health care provider every week or two until you go into labour.

GETTING TO APPOINTMENTS

In some provinces and territories, if you live in a remote area and must travel to an urban centre for special medical care, you may be able to apply for a government travel grant. Ask your health care provider if this applies to you.

Some First Nations, and Inuit may have access to Health Canada's Non-Insured Health Benefits Program to help pay for medical transportation and other health care costs during pregnancy and childbirth. To learn more about this program, contact your Non-Insured Health Benefits Regional Office or visit their website at www.hc-sc.gc.ca/fniah-spnia/ nihb-ssna/index-eng.php.

WHAT IS MY DUE DATE?

The Big Day—your due date—is calculated by counting 9 calendar months, plus 7 days from the first day of your last menstrual period. For women with regular cycles this easy method is surprisingly accurate. But an ultrasound is the most accurate way to calculate the due date.

About 85% of babies are born within a week of (before or after) their due date.

Your first prenatal visit

You should book your first prenatal visit as soon as you learn you are pregnant. At your first visit expect to have a complete check-up. It may include a pregnancy test to confirm your pregnancy and an internal physical exam of your reproductive organs and pelvis.

You will be asked to provide details about your medical history and other births and pregnancies. You will be asked if your immunizations are up-to-date. If you saw your health care provider when you were planning to get pregnant, you may review health concerns that you discussed then. During this visit, your health care provider will also calculate your due date. This is usually done by counting from the first day of your last menstrual period. That's why it's helpful if you know this date for your first visit.

Your health care provider knows how important it is for you to be well-informed about your pregnancy and your developing baby. It is also a good time to have a discussion about how to prepare for breastfeeding. Prenatal visits may not cover every topic. It is helpful to read materials such as this handbook and attend prenatal classes.

About weight gain

Weight gain during pregnancy is necessary. It supports the growth of the fetus and the placenta, as well as changes in your body, such as an increased volume of blood and fluid, larger breast size, and some storage of fat. Weight and fat are sensitive topics for most women. In pregnancy the goal is simple: to accept whatever weight you start at and work with it so that you have the healthiest possible pregnancy and your baby the healthiest start in life.

The amount of weight gain that is right for you depends on your BMI before you got pregnant. BMI stands for "body mass index." Your health care provider can calculate your BMI based on your height and weight and let you know if you are overweight, underweight, or at the ideal weight. You can also calculate your BMI using this formula: BMI = weight(kg)/height(m)^2. The BMI categories are not intended for use by those under 18 years of age or for pregnant or breastfeeding women. Weight gain is usually slow during the first 3 months. Most weight gain will happen in the second and third trimesters. Gaining weight at a steady pace is a sign of a healthy pregnancy. Talk to your health care provider if you are gaining a lot more than 0.4 kg (1 lb) a week or a lot less.

Dietitians of Canada has an online tool to measure your BMI at www.dietitians.ca/Your-Health/Assess-Yourself/Assess-Your-BMI/BMI-Adult.aspx.

MEET YOUR ENERGY NEEDS

Pregnant women may not need to increase calories during the first trimester, but you will need to eat a little more in the second and third trimesters. You don't want to "eat for two"—but you should eat to satisfy your appetite—ideally, an extra two to three Food Guide servings. A healthy snack combines at least two of the four food groups (such as half a sandwich—try turkey with tomato, made with whole grain bread—and a glass of milk).

How much weight should a woman gain during pregnancy?				
Pre-pregnancy BMI	Mean rate of weight gain in second and third trimesters		Recommended total weight gain	
	kg/week	lbs/week	kg	lbs
BMI < 18.5	0.5	1	12.5 to 18	28 to 40
BMI 18.5 to 24.9	0.4	1	11.5 to 16	25 to 35
BMI 25.0 to 29.9	0.3	0.6	7 to 11.5	15 to 25
BMI ≥ 30.0*	0.2	0.5	5 to 9	11 to 20

Women with a BMI over 35 should talk to their health care provider about appropriate weight gain during pregnancy.

Source: J Obstet Gynaecol Can 2016; 38(6):508e554.

ARE YOU SOMEONE WHO NEEDS MORE CALORIES?

☐ *I am having more than one baby.*

☐ *I am a teenager.*

☐ *I am very physically active.*

☐ *I have had a baby with low birth weight (baby weighed less than 2.5 kg/5.5 lbs at birth).*

☐ *I am thin (underweight).*

☐ *I am going through a lot of emotional stress.*

If you checked off any of these boxes, speak to your health care provider. You might need more calories during pregnancy.

Be aware of your special need for iron, folic acid, and essential fatty acids.

Refer to the nutrition section in Chapter One.

Women who gain too much weight during pregnancy are more likely to have large babies and children who are overweight. They also have a higher risk for complications during pregnancy, such as gestational diabetes and pre-eclampsia. However, not gaining enough weight during pregnancy can also be a problem. This applies especially to young adolescent women (teenagers) who still have their own growing to do.

If you do gain more weight than recommended during pregnancy, it is advised that you do not try to lose weight while you are pregnant. Just stick to the weekly weight gain targets recommended by your health care provider until the birth.

To learn more about where your gained weight goes in supporting your baby, visit Health Canada's website at www.hc-sc.gc.ca/fn-an/nutrition/prenatal/hwgdp-ppspg-eng.php.

For more details about nutrition and pregnancy, see Chapter One.

About vitamin supplements

Take a multivitamin daily before and during your pregnancy.

If you are not already taking a multivitamin containing folic acid and iron, now is the next best time to start. A daily multivitamin provides important vitamins and minerals, including folic acid and iron. Some women need more folic acid or iron. It is important to take only what is recommended by your health care provider. Check the label on your multivitamin to make sure it contains what and how much your health care provider recommends. Not all prenatal vitamins and multivitamins are the same. Folic acid helps cells develop and reduces the risk of some birth defects. Folic acid is important early in pregnancy. A folic acid supplement (0.4 mg), in addition to a diet rich in folic acid, is recommended for:

- All women who could get pregnant
- All pregnant women
- All breastfeeding women

The recommended total daily intake of iron for pregnant women is 27 mg. Pregnant women often have difficulty getting enough iron from their food. A daily multivitamin with 16–20 mg of iron can help you get enough. Talk to your health care provider if you have side effects from the multivitamin, such as indigestion or constipation.

Discussing your pregnancy

Talk honestly with your health care team during your pregnancy. Your overall well-being is an important aspect of a healthy pregnancy. Here are some things that are important to discuss with your team:

- Tell them how you feel about the pregnancy.
- Talk about your partner and the role he or she may play during the pregnancy.
- Tell them if you feel safe or unsafe, loved or not loved, and about the kind of bond you have with your partner.
- Explain how your family and friends feel about this pregnancy.
- Find out where you can go for prenatal classes and what you can do to keep you and your baby as healthy as possible.

Think about taking this journal with you each time you see your health care provider. We have left space at the end of the chapter so you can write down questions for your health care provider as well as the answers.

WHY DO I NEED TO SEE MY HEALTH CARE PROVIDER WHEN I FEEL FINE?

Prenatal care is the term for the medical care you receive before your baby is born. Almost 90% of pregnancies and babies are healthy, and studies show that women who have regular prenatal care have healthier pregnancies and healthier babies. To help ensure you have a healthy pregnancy, make an appointment as soon as you know you are pregnant.

Also, getting to know your health care provider—especially at an early stage—will make it easier for you to share your concerns and ask your questions openly. Regular check-ups also make it easier for your health care provider to spot any possible problems early on so you can take steps to try to prevent any health concerns.

"GOING IT ALONE"

Perhaps you are pregnant and don't have a partner for support. Other people can help, including your family and friends. Hopefully you can create a support team and find people you can trust and talk with. You might find it helpful to do the following:

- *Make a list of the things you need help with. Ask friends and family to help you.*

- *Early on, ask someone you trust to be your birth "partner."*

- *Take someone with you to your health care provider appointments, scans, or tests.*

- *Go shopping with friends or family to buy the things you need for the baby . . . and for yourself!*

- *Find out if there is a drop-in program in your community for pregnant women or new parents.*

If you are a teenager, talk to a health care provider or other community resource person about the support your community may offer.

Our heritage and our health

Our heritage affects not only our birth traditions and customs but also our individual risk of certain medical complications. This means that women may have very different cultural and medical wants and needs during pregnancy and childbirth, depending on their ancestry. If your health care provider is not familiar with your heritage, he or she may welcome the opportunity to learn more from you and take your heritage into account when providing your prenatal care. Your provider will look out for any particular medical complications that you may be more prone to, such as diabetes, or that may affect your baby, such as diabetes or Tay Sachs.

You are expecting twins . . . or more!

If you know you will be giving birth to twins, triplets, or more, you are not alone! In Canada, 3.5% of births are multiples, and that number is rising. You might be feeling excited and overwhelmed at the same time. How will you cope? What kind of care will you and your babies need? There will be many joys, but what are the risks?

You will need special health care and support while you are pregnant. There are some complications that are more common with multiples, such as having a preterm birth (see page 99).

Early and regular health care and support are important to help you avoid problems with your pregnancy and birth. Your health care provider will likely recommend that you have appointments with a specialist (such as an obstetrician or a doctor who specializes in multiple births).

Learn more about multiple births from Multiple Births Canada's website at www.multiplebirthscanada.org.

Prenatal classes and preparing for birth

Prenatal education programs are an important part of your care and support during pregnancy. Prenatal education can be a series of classes, either online or in-person, provided for pregnant women, their partner, and/or support people.

Prenatal education can:

- Provide the information and skills you need to have a healthy pregnancy and baby
- Promote a positive birthing experience
- Prepare you for parenting

LIST OF REGISTRATION AND CONTACT INFORMATION, DATES, LOCATIONS, AND TIMES FOR PRENATAL CLASSES

- Prepare you for breastfeeding
- Enhance communication between partners about pregnancy and parenting

Prenatal classes vary and may cover topics such as nutrition and exercise during pregnancy, discomforts and changes during pregnancy, preterm labour, labour and birth, pain management during labour, breastfeeding, and taking care of yourself and new baby after the birth. Parenting, recovery, and sex after birth and normal infant development may also be covered.

Prenatal classes include partners, support people, and sometimes even children. When partners go to classes, they can learn about their changing relationship and their new role as parents. Children can learn to prepare for the birth of a new brother or sister.

Some prenatal classes are designed for different ethnic or cultural backgrounds. They may be offered in languages other than English or French. Other classes focus on the needs of teens or the needs of Indigenous communities or new Canadians. Ask your health care provider about what exists in your community and how you can register for classes.

Travel during pregnancy

Travel is easiest before your 20th week of pregnancy. After 20 weeks, think about where you will travel, how you will travel, how far you will travel, and the length of time you will be away from home.

A quick flight is different from a long car ride across the country or a trip overseas. Before you plan a trip, you should always talk to your health care provider. Carry all the basic details about your pregnancy with you. This includes your blood type and the results of your latest ultrasound. This information may help you in case of an emergency or if you are faced with something you did not plan.

Airlines prefer that you do not travel in late pregnancy, and you may require a note from your health care provider to travel. Check with your airline and be sure that you have travel insurance to cover both yourself and your baby should you go into labour while away from home.

International travel

It is important to look at the Public Health Agency of Canada website on travel health and safety. The site contains a list of diseases, risks, and travel notices. Visit www.phac-aspc.gc.ca/tmp-pmv/info/index-eng.php.

Talk with your health care provider at least a month before you travel internationally about any vaccines you might need. The Government of Canada has information about immunization for pregnant and breastfeeding women. Visit www.healthycanadians.gc.ca/healthy-living-vie-saine/immunization-immunisation/pregnancy-grossesse/index-eng.php#a2.

Zika virus

Zika is a mosquito-borne disease that is present in many warm climate countries (for a full list consult Health Canada's travel health notices at www.travel.gc.ca/travelling/health-safety/travel-health-notices). It can cause serious birth defects, most notably a brain malformation called *microcephaly*. Pregnant women and those considering becoming pregnant should discuss travel plans with their health care provider to assess their risk and consider postponing travel to areas that may have Zika virus. If travel cannot be postponed, follow strict mosquito bite prevention measures.

Women who want to get pregnant should wait *at least 6 months* after their return from areas that may have Zika virus, before trying to conceive. Men returning from a Zika area may pass the virus through sexual transmission and should use barrier precautions (condoms) for 6 months. Consult your health care provider for up-to-date advice.

For more information on travelling while pregnant, visit www.travel.gc.ca/travelling/health-safety/travelling-pregnant.

Sex during pregnancy

Many pregnant women feel a change in their levels of sexual desire: in some women it goes up and in others it goes down. There is no right and wrong. Men can have concerns, or different feelings about sex in pregnancy; some facts may help.

In most cases, having intercourse will not harm you or the pregnancy in any way. However, your health care provider may tell you to avoid or limit intercourse if you have:

- An infection
- Bleeding
- Ruptured membranes
- Some pregnancy complications

If you are at risk of a sexually transmitted infection, continue to use condoms to protect you and your growing baby.

Some couples feel closer during this special time and continue to enjoy sex until just before their baby is due. Other couples feel their relationship is strained by all the changes taking place. They find that sex is not as fulfilling during pregnancy. Your partner may be worried that having sex could harm the baby. If either of you is uncomfortable about sexual relations, make time for other kinds of physical touch. You can cuddle with each other, hold hands, discuss how you feel, give or get a massage, or take a bath together.

If you are comfortable with the idea, you can explore other options such as masturbation and oral sex. Just a warning about oral sex: ask your partner to be very careful **not to blow any air into your vagina.** Doing this could force air into your bloodstream, which could be fatal to both you and your baby.

Exercise during pregnancy

Whether or not you are pregnant, exercise is good for you. It is important not to overdo the activities you choose. We suggest you try different workouts that can be part of your daily routine: aerobic exercise (with caution; see the next section), strength training, yoga, and tai chi.

The Physical Activity Resource Centre (PARC) has a great resource called "Active Pregnancy" that can be downloaded at www.ophea. net/active-pregnancy. It provides guidelines to ensure pregnant women are exercising safely.

Aerobic exercise

Exercise that makes your heart beat faster than when you are resting is called *aerobic exercise.* This kind of exercise uses the large muscle groups. It includes walking, running, swimming, stationary bikes, low-impact aerobics, cross-country skiing, aquafit, or team sports.

If you were active before you became pregnant, you can likely continue with the same or a slightly lower level of activity. Discuss your exercise plans with your health care provider early in your pregnancy to make sure you do not have any health problems that

SLEEPING DURING PREGNANCY: IT IS THE WHAT NOT THE HOW

You may have come across advice to sleep on your left side; however, it is not easy to change your natural sleep position, and the reported risks of other sleep positions are very rare. The most important thing is that you get a good night's sleep. (See page 93, "Feeling dizzy when you are flat on your back," in Chapter Three.)

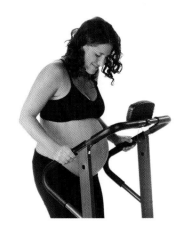

WHEN IS IT NOT SAFE TO
EXERCISE?

*As you read this list, check off any of
the statements that are true for you.*

☐ *I have heart problems.*

☐ *I have a serious lung condition
and/or breathing problems.*

☐ *I have high blood pressure.*

☐ *I had bleeding from my vagina
during this pregnancy.*

☐ *I have low levels of iron in my
blood (anemia).*

☐ *I am carrying more than one
baby.*

☐ *I have problems controlling my
blood sugar levels.*

☐ *I have concerns about my
blood sugar levels.*

☐ *My health care provider told me
the fetus is too small for its age.*

☐ *I am at high risk for preterm
labour.*

☐ *I am very underweight or have
been diagnosed with an eating
disorder.*

☐ *I suspect I have a rupture of
the membranes.*

*If you have ticked any of these boxes,
ask your health care provider how
much exercise you can engage in.*

would make vigorous exercise risky. Most women who are runners can continue to run when they are pregnant without harm to their growing baby. If you feel pain in the pubic region, this is a sign that your body is not adapting well to running and you should stop.

Exercise is good for you and your baby. If you haven't been physically active at least two to three times per week before becoming pregnant, you should wait until your second trimester, when the risks and discomforts of pregnancy are at their lowest, to begin exercising and only after you discuss your choices with your health care provider. Walking is always encouraged, regardless of previous activity level unless your health care provider has advised you to limit activity.

Your baby is not able to cool down if you get overheated with exercise. During pregnancy, it is not advisable to exhaust yourself. If you are worried about exercising too hard, try the "talk test." You should always be able to talk during your workout. Otherwise, lower your level of effort.

Once your health care provider says it's okay to exercise, begin to do so. Walk, swim, or join a fitness class. Some classes are designed just for pregnant women and new mothers. If you are part of a regular aerobics class, talk to your teacher about what you might need to avoid (routines that are high-impact or that put stress on your lower back).

Strength training

Building and maintaining muscle mass is an important part of any exercise program. But be cautious! Remember to breathe regularly during each part of the weight-training motion. Talk to your health care provider before you begin or continue a weight-training program.

Rules to follow when you exercise

Consult with your health care provider before beginning or changing physical activity.

Always warm up muscles before activity and stretch after your activity. Never stretch a cold muscle.

Aerobic exercise

- During pregnancy, you should limit your aerobic exercise sessions to 30 to 40 minutes, including the warm-up and cool-down. Warm-up is a time for your body to adjust to an increased heart rate. It is best to begin your activity slowly, at low intensity, and to gradually increase your movement for 5 to 8 minutes. For runners, this means your first 5 to 8 minutes should be variable speed walking. Cool-down will take another 5 to 8 minutes and should consist of slowing your body down by doing some deep breathing and slow stretching.
- Take rest breaks when you feel you need them. Keep your heart rate at the low end of the target heart rate for women your age. Check yourself by using the talk test.
- Drink one glass of water every exercise session. You can drink it 30 minutes before or right after the session. The important thing is to keep well hydrated every day and not just when you are exercising.
- Be careful when you are doing sports that require balance and coordination. During your pregnancy, your centre of gravity will be constantly changing.
- Avoid contact sports and any activity that might make you fall or be hit. This includes downhill skiing, mountain climbing, floor hockey, water skiing, horseback riding, cycling, gymnastics, and soccer.

AM I EXERCISING TOO HARD?

Check off any of the statements that are true for you.

- ☐ *I feel exhausted during my workout.*
- ☐ *I feel very hot and dehydrated when I exercise.*
- ☐ *I have trouble talking when I exercise.*
- ☐ *I have chest pain, jaw pain, or unexplained arm pain.*
- ☐ *I feel dizzy during or after exercise.*

If you ticked any of these boxes, you are overexerting yourself during your workout. It would be best to reduce the level of your exercise routine and talk to your health care provider.

THE TALK TEST

You should always be able to carry on a conversation when you are exercising. If you cannot, you are working too hard. If you can, you are doing great.

EXERCISE SAFETY CONSIDERATIONS

- *Avoid exercise in warm or humid environments, especially during the first trimester.*

- *Avoid straining while you are holding your breath.*

- *Eat well and stay hydrated. Drink liquids before and after exercise.*

- *Avoid exercising while lying on your back past the fourth month of pregnancy.*

- *Avoid activities that involve physical contact or danger of falling.*

- *Know your limits. Pregnancy is not a good time to train for an athletic competition.*

- *Know the reasons to stop exercise and consult a qualified health care provider immediately if they occur.*

Source: Physical Activity Readiness Medical Examination for Pregnancy (PARmed-X for Pregnancy) © 2002. Used with permission from the Canadian Society for Exercise Physiology www.csep.ca. If you have Internet access, you can download the complete guideline questionnaire from www.csep.ca/cmfiles/ publications/parq/parmed-xpreg.pdf.

Strength training

Avoid any exercise that causes you to hold your breath and bear down at the same time, such as heavy weight–lifting routines.

After the fourth month of pregnancy, you should change your abdominal exercises. Stop lying on your back when you do them. Instead, lie on your side or do the exercise while you are standing.

Avoid stretching ligaments and tendons too much. This becomes more likely because they may be more flexible because of pregnancy hormones. Prenatal yoga is considered safe and effective in helping to feel more toned and flexible. It will also help reduce stress and help you to relax during pregnancy. Pilates has not been studied in pregnancy. If qualified instructors know you are pregnant, they will suggest ways for you to adjust so you can be safe.

The most important muscles to tone when you are pregnant are the pelvic muscles. (See page 59 to learn about Kegel exercises.) They help develop pelvic and core strength. Core stability takes some stress off the pelvic floor and prevents your body from using your pelvic muscles too much.

At the gym or fitness centre

Avoid exercises that strain your lower back. Always maintain good posture.

Also, be careful of your body temperature, especially if exercising in warm and humid environments (either indoors or outdoors). Warm weather exercise should be balanced by drinking lots of fluids. Avoid hot tubs, saunas, and steam rooms.

Kegel exercises strengthen your core and pelvic floor muscles

Kegel exercises provide strength training for the muscles that surround your pelvic floor. Kegel exercises will also help prevent a flow of urine when you cough, lift, or laugh. By learning this routine, you will develop a good habit for life. It helps you get back in shape after childbirth. It will also help you prevent urine flow problems later in life.

Learn how to do pelvic exercises properly. A physiotherapist who specializes in pelvic floor rehabilitation can help with this.

1. Sit or stand comfortably. Relax.
2. Find your pelvic muscle. Imagine that you are trying to hold back urine or a bowel movement. Squeeze the muscles you would use to do that.
3. Tighten the muscles for 5 to 10 seconds.
4. Do not hold your breath—breathe normally.
5. Do not tighten your stomach or buttocks—keep them relaxed.
6. Now relax the muscles for about 10 seconds.
7. Repeat the squeeze-hold-relax routine 12 to 20 times.

What are these tests for?

When you go to your first prenatal visit, your health care provider will recommend routine laboratory tests. These help to find or predict risks to your health and the health of your baby.

PELVIC TILTS MAY HELP TO RELIEVE YOUR BACKACHE

Do this simple exercise two or three times a day. It will strengthen your abdominal muscles and take some pressure off your aching back.

- *Lie on the floor and relax your back.*

- *Exhale and pull your buttocks forward, pulling your pubic bone upward while keeping your lower back on the floor.*

- *Hold this position for a count of three, then inhale and relax.*

- *Repeat five times.*

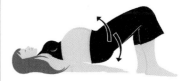

 Pelvic tilt

Blood and other tests

The tests you will be offered depend on your medical history. Common tests include the following:

- **Blood type and antibodies:** to identify your blood group and rhesus (Rh) factor. This test also looks for any unusual antibodies in your blood. (See page 63, "Blood types and Rh factors.")
- **Hemoglobin:** to check your blood to make sure it can carry enough iron and oxygen. (See page 30, "Anemia and iron.")
- **Hepatitis B surface antigens:** to see if you have been exposed to hepatitis B. (See page 68, "Hepatitis B.")
- **HIV:** to check whether you have been exposed to HIV, the virus that causes AIDS. (See page 70, "HIV and AIDS.")
- **Rubella titre:** to see if you have immunity to rubella (German measles). (See page 67, "Rubella (German measles) or varicella (chicken pox).")
- **Varicella (chicken pox):** to see if you have immunity to this virus. If you had chicken pox when you were younger, your body will have immunity and you will not need to have this test. (See page 67, "Rubella (German measles) or varicella (chicken pox).")
- **Syphilis screening:** to see if you have been exposed to syphilis, a sexually transmitted infection.
- **Pap test:** to check for cancer of the cervix or abnormal cells that could lead to cancer.
- **Urine test:** to check sugar levels, which could be a sign of diabetes, and protein levels, which could indicate pre-eclampsia, a type of high blood pressure in pregnancy. This test is also used to find out if you have a urinary tract infection. This kind of infection can be treated, but without treatment, your risk of preterm labour rises.

Genetic screening

Medicine today gives us new ways to understand and diagnose hereditary problems passed through the genes of the mother and/or father as well as birth defects in the baby that have different causes. The following can increase the risk of a birth defect:

- A family member has a birth defect
- Older mother or father
- Use of certain medicines, street drugs, and alcohol (see pages 36 to 38)
- Some diseases in early pregnancy

Some defects or conditions cannot be explained but affect the baby's development.

When a health problem is hereditary, this means it is passed through the genes of the mother or the father to a child, the same way as eye colour or hair colour. Sometimes, these kinds of health problems can be found using special tests that will require a referral to a genetic specialist.

At your first prenatal visit, your health care provider will talk about:

- Blood-screening tests for certain genetic disorders
- Ultrasound

The majority of pregnancies in Canada result in the birth of a healthy baby. Knowing about problems or risk before the baby is born can help families and health care providers plan for the future and for any special medical care or treatment that might be needed.

In Canada, genetic screening is offered to all women. You can decide whether or not you want genetic screening. Screening options vary by community.

GENETIC DISORDERS AND BIRTH DEFECTS

Before pregnancy or early in pregnancy it is important to learn as much as possible about your family's medical history. You should also find out about the medical history of the birth father's family. You should let your health care provider know if either family has any of the following conditions:

- ☐ *Anencephaly*
- ☐ *Born with extra fingers or toes*
- ☐ *Cleft palate*
- ☐ *Clubfoot*
- ☐ *Congenital heart defect*
- ☐ *Cystic fibrosis*
- ☐ *Down syndrome*
- ☐ *Fragile X syndrome*
- ☐ *Hemophilia*
- ☐ *Huntington's disease*
- ☐ *Muscular dystrophy*
- ☐ *Sickle cell disease*
- ☐ *Spina bifida*
- ☐ *Tay-Sachs disease*
- ☐ *Thalassemia*
- ☐ *Other _____*

In addition to the standard screening, there are now highly sensitive blood tests that analyze DNA from the baby that is in the mother's circulation, often referred to as non-invasive prenatal testing, or cell-free DNA testing. If the results are abnormal, additional tests are required to see if there is actually a health concern for your baby. The costs of these tests may be covered in some cases but often are not.

Testing may be done using blood tests or ultrasound or both combined. Other tests may be recommended if it seems you are at higher risk of giving birth to a child with certain types of conditions or medical problems.

Tests are important. Some tests are routine—recommended for all pregnancies. Others are recommended only when certain details are needed to identify a condition.

No test is 100% accurate and no single test covers all possible conditions. There are risks as well as benefits to testing. For example, some tests need a tissue or fluid sample from the baby. This may involve inserting a needle into your abdomen to take the sample. Doing this is common, but there is a small risk. Your health care provider will discuss the need for certain tests, any risks involved, and then he or she will make a recommendation. In the end, you will be the one who decides whether to have a test or not.

Tests that check your baby's health before birth

There are many types of tests that can check your baby's development. Some are offered to all women early on and throughout the pregnancy (such as ultrasound). Other tests, such as amniocentesis, are offered only if there is a specific concern or possible risk. Some of these special tests can pose a small risk to the mother and/or the baby. Your health care provider will not suggest a test unless you need it.

Blood types and Rh factors

It is important to know what your blood type is when you are pregnant. This can be determined with one of the tests offered during your first prenatal visit. Although you likely won't need a blood transfusion during your pregnancy or during the birth, if you do, the health care providers need to know what type of blood to give you. There are four blood types: O, A, B, and AB. Type O blood is the most common type in North America.

You may have also heard of "Rh factor" in people's blood. Everyone's blood is either Rh positive or Rh negative.

A baby's blood type and Rh factor depend on his or her parents' blood types and Rh factors—just like eye colour, skin colour, or hair colour. A baby may have the blood type and the Rh factor of either parent or a combination of both parents' types and factors.

Only 15% of the population is Rh negative. Problems may occur if the mother is Rh negative and the baby is Rh positive. In Rh disease, antibodies formed in the mother can cross to the baby's circulation and attack the baby's blood cells, causing severe anemia. At one time, this led to Rh disease and caused serious illnesses or death of the baby. Now that we can identify who is at risk and prevent Rh disease, it has become very rare. If your blood test shows that your baby is at risk of Rh disease, it will be recommended that you receive Rh-immune globulin (RhIg) between the 28th and 32nd weeks of pregnancy and again after your baby's birth or at any time during pregnancy if bleeding occurs. This will protect your baby from Rh disease.

If you are Rh negative, your baby is at risk of Rh disease. Rh-immune globulin will be recommended regardless if it is very early in pregnancy that ends in miscarriage or abortion or an ongoing pregnancy. If you do have bleeding in early pregnancy, be sure to let your health care provider know that you are Rh negative. If you carry an Rh positive baby, your body can be sensitized and make Rh antibodies that can harm a future pregnancy.

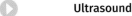

Ultrasound

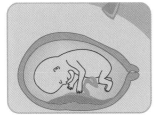

Ultrasound

Most people have heard about ultrasound. One of the purposes of ultrasound is to confirm your baby's due date. It is recommended that you have an ultrasound test at least once, usually at 18 weeks of pregnancy and, if possible, prior to 23 weeks. Dating is more accurate on the earlier ultrasound. By 23 weeks, the baby is sufficiently well formed that the ultrasonographer can check on your baby's health and growth, if there is a concern.

The test uses sound waves to create a picture of your baby on a computer screen. An ultrasound takes pictures by sending sound waves that travel safely into your body, and these waves "bounce back" and are turned into images. You, your family, and your health care providers will be able to see a real-time, shaded image of the baby. Ultrasound is used for these reasons:

- To check the age of the baby and estimate due date
- To see the baby's position
- To check the baby's growth and well-being
- To find out where the placenta is attached to the uterus
- To see if there is more than one baby
- To check for some abnormalities

Ultrasound

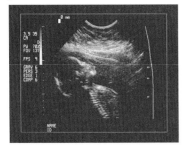

The ultrasound technician will apply gel to your belly. This gel helps a small hand-held device called a *transducer* (which sends the sound waves) to move easily over your skin. You will not hear the sound wave, but you might feel light pressure on your belly, and you will not feel any pain. Most ultrasound exams last about 30 minutes. If your health care provider has asked for more details from an ultrasound, the test could take longer.

Before you go for an ultrasound, you will learn how to prepare and where to go for the test. Sometimes, you will be told to arrive with a full bladder. This helps the sound waves travel through the skin and tissues to get a better picture of your baby.

Some women might need to have the ultrasound done through the vagina. The ultrasound technician uses a special transducer that is inserted into the vagina. This should not hurt but may be uncomfortable.

Testing for genetic disorders

Integrated prenatal screening (IPS)

This refers to blood tests that measure substances in the mother's blood called *markers*. High levels of these markers may mean the baby is at risk for certain conditions. Positive results only indicate a higher risk. Other tests will need to be done to confirm this. If offered in your area, your health care provider will give you reading material to help you decide whether or not to have this testing done.

Nuchal translucency

This special type of ultrasound is offered in some areas to screen for Down syndrome. The test is offered between the 11th and 14th week of pregnancy. It measures the thickness of the layer of fluid at the back of the baby's neck. If the layer is thicker than average, this means a higher likelihood of Down syndrome. A woman will then be offered a test called *amniocentesis*. Both amniocentesis and genetic blood tests may be used to make a more accurate diagnosis regarding certain genetic disorders.

Prenatal cell-free DNA screening or NIPT (non-invasive prenatal testing)

NIPT is a non-invasive blood test that detects conditions that are caused by an abnormal chromosome. The testing is done on a mother's blood sample and looks for fetal DNA in the mother's circulation.

It is a very accurate screening test and can be done after 10 weeks of pregnancy, but it is only a screening test, so abnormal results always have to be confirmed by further testing using chorionic villus sampling or amniocentesis.

This test is available in Canada and may be covered by health care plans in certain provinces or if you have particular risk factors.

Chorionic villus sampling (CVS)

This is another test for genetic-related disorders. It is not a routine test, but it is offered when there is a higher suspicion of a genetic problem and is usually covered by insurance. It is done between the 10th and 12th weeks of pregnancy. The doctor uses an ultrasound to pass a small needle through the cervix or the abdomen into the placenta to take a sample of special cells (chorionic villi).

Amniocentesis

A number of genetic or inherited disorders can be identified by taking a sample of the amniotic fluid that surrounds the baby. This test is offered after the 14th week of pregnancy and is usually covered by insurance. A fine needle is inserted into the uterus via the abdomen. Ultrasound helps the doctor find a safe place to insert the needle. It may take up to 4 weeks to get the full results of this test.

Tay-Sachs screening

Tay-Sachs disease is a rare disorder passed from parents to the child. Generally, a baby will show symptoms at about 6 months old. The enzyme that helps break down fatty substances is absent, and toxic levels build in the brain and nerve cells. The disease results in loss of body function, leading to blindness, paralysis, and death. Unfortunately there is no cure.

Tay-Sachs disease occurs most often among people whose ancestors come from Eastern and Central European Jewish communities

Chorionic villus sampling

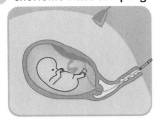

Amniocentesis

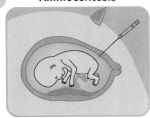

(Ashkenazi Jews), from certain communities in Quebec, the Old Order Amish community in Pennsylvania, and from the Cajun community of Louisiana. A child who inherits the gene from both parents develops Tay-Sachs disease. Genetic screening is offered to the pregnant woman and is usually covered by insurance. Experts recommend both parents be tested.

Infectious diseases to be aware of in pregnancy

Fifth disease

Fifth disease is a common viral illness among children. It is caused by parvovirus B19. It is usually very mild and appears in children as a red rash on the face, trunk, arms, and legs. If you are pregnant and you often spend time with young children, you may come in contact with the disease. However, more than half of women have been infected once and are now immune. Women who get the infection may have fever, a rash, and joint pain. Most women have no symptoms and no serious complications. In very rare cases, the virus can infect an unborn baby and cause illness or death.

If a pregnant woman is exposed to or shows signs of a parvovirus infection, she should have her blood tested to see if she is already immune. Certain women are at a higher risk of being exposed. They include daycare workers, school teachers, and mothers of young children. However, there is no proof that women reduce their risk of infection by leaving work. If you spend a lot of time with children, washing your hands frequently helps to decrease your chance of infection. If you are pregnant and think you may have been exposed to this virus, talk to your health care provider.

Rubella (German measles) or varicella (chicken pox)

Both rubella and varicella can cause serious problems for a growing baby. It is best to make sure that you are immune before

AM I AT RISK FOR HEPATITIS B?

☐ *I had a blood transfusion or blood products for a clotting disorder.*

☐ *I have had more than one sexual partner.*

☐ *I have injected drugs.*

☐ *I shared needles when I injected drugs.*

☐ *I handled blood or blood products at my job.*

☐ *I was born in Asia.*

If you checked one or more boxes, you are at higher risk of having hepatitis B.

If you have hepatitis B, a vaccine can protect your baby.

you get pregnant. If you are vaccinated before becoming pregnant, wait at least 1 month before you try to conceive.

If you are not immune to either rubella or varicella and you are pregnant, your health care provider will discuss the risks and options with you. Pregnant women should avoid being immunized against rubella or varicella; however, you may be vaccinated after giving birth.

Hepatitis B

There are several types of hepatitis, a viral infection that affects the liver. Hepatitis B is the type that can affect babies during pregnancy. It can be spread during sexual contact or passed to a baby during childbirth. It is the most serious type of hepatitis during pregnancy. One in every 250 people has this disease. It is more common in people who have recently moved to Canada from Asia.

Many people with hepatitis B have no symptoms and do not even know they have it. They are called *chronic carriers,* and they can pass hepatitis B on to other people. A small percentage of chronic carriers will develop a very serious liver disease that can cause death.

Without treatment, about 50% of babies born to mothers who test positive for hepatitis B will be infected. This usually happens during birth or while breastfeeding. Without treatment, many of these babies will become chronic carriers and a few may develop long-term health problems.

Babies born to mothers who test positive for hepatitis B can be treated soon after birth. They will receive both the hepatitis B immune globulin and the hepatitis B vaccine. With treatment, 95% of these babies will not be infected, nor will they become carriers.

Herpes

Herpes is a virus that causes cold sores and genital infections. At least 10% of people have one of the two forms called *herpes simplex virus (HSV)*. Although the virus is not life-threatening to adults, it can spread easily between sexual partners and can be painful and troublesome. Pregnant women should know about herpes because the virus can infect the baby during birth and cause serious harm.

The most common type of herpes infection is HSV-1, the type that most often causes cold sores on the face, mostly on the lips. The other, HSV-2, most often occurs on the sex organs (genitals) of men and women. Either type can infect the face or genitals.

What are the risks of herpes to your baby?

The greatest danger to your baby comes during birth. The baby may get neonatal herpes if you have herpes. Although this is rare, it is also life-threatening and can create skin, eye, and mouth infections and damage to the baby's central nervous system and other internal organs.

What should you do if you or your partner has herpes?

You should tell your health care provider if you suspect that you or your partner has either type of herpes. You should avoid sexual intercourse and oral sex with partners who have, or you suspect may have, an active herpes outbreak.

Having a genital herpes infection for the first time, near the time of birth, is the greatest risk to your baby. If you have genital herpes, your health care provider may suggest you take antiviral medications during the last 4 weeks of pregnancy. This will decrease the chance of an outbreak at birth. If you have an outbreak at the time of birth, then a caesarean birth probably will be recommended.

DO I HAVE A LIFESTYLE THAT
PUTS ME AT RISK FOR SEXUALLY
TRANSMITTED INFECTIONS (STIs)?

☐ *I have had many sexual partners.*

☐ *I have had sex with many partners, some of whom did not wear a condom.*

☐ *I use street drugs.*

☐ *I inject street drugs.*

☐ *I have a drinking problem.*

If you agree with any of these statements, you are at higher risk of getting a sexually transmitted infection. You should be tested for STIs (including HIV).

HIV and AIDS

Human immunodeficiency virus (HIV) is found in an infected person's body fluids. This includes semen, blood, vaginal fluids, and breast milk. HIV causes infections and diseases that harm a person's immune and nervous systems. HIV can lead to acquired immune deficiency syndrome (AIDS)—the name of the disease caused by HIV that can lead to death.

Symptoms of HIV may take 5 years or more to appear. Many people with HIV do not know they have it. But HIV can be found in a simple blood test. The most common way for the virus to spread from an infected person to a non-infected person is during sex. However, the virus can also enter a person's bloodstream through a needle that carries the virus. You will be at risk if you share needles with an HIV-positive intravenous drug user. It is very rare to get an HIV infection from a blood transfusion. In Canada, the blood supply is carefully screened for HIV.

You can reduce your chances of getting HIV by doing the following:

- Asking questions about your partner's sexual past before you have sexual contact
- Limiting the number of sexual partners you have

You can protect yourself from HIV, in a new relationship, by using a condom for at least 6 months. After two negative HIV tests by both people, it is probably safe to stop using condoms—as long as you have also been tested for other sexually transmitted infections and neither of you has other sexual partners. If you use injection drugs, never share needles.

The number of women who have HIV is rising. A pregnant woman can pass the virus on to her child during pregnancy, childbirth, or while breastfeeding. Transmission of the virus is more likely during mixed breastfeeding and formula feeding than during exclusive breastfeeding. Women who know they are HIV positive can greatly reduce their baby's chance of getting the virus (down to 1%) if they receive treatment throughout pregnancy and during labour and if the baby gets treatment during the first 6 weeks of life.

That is why every woman who is pregnant, or thinking about getting pregnant, should be tested for HIV. All pregnant women in Canada are offered HIV testing during pregnancy for free.

About dental health

The hormonal changes that come with pregnancy can also affect your teeth and gums. Some women notice that their gums become swollen or may even bleed. It's an important time to keep any regular dental appointments and to brush and floss regularly. Pregnant women with tooth decay and gum disease may be at increased risk for preterm birth. Talk to your dentist if you have questions or problems. If you do not have access to a dentist, talk to a community health nurse.

Common discomforts in early pregnancy

Nausea and vomiting

We still do not know what causes "morning sickness." It happens most often during the first 3 or 4 months of pregnancy, but sometimes it can last longer. You may feel nauseated during the day or night and when your stomach is empty.

For most women, the nausea will ease up a bit at some point during the day. This gives them a chance to feel hungry again and to eat food that will stay in their stomachs. However, 1% of pregnant

---

DENTAL HEALTH IS IMPORTANT IN PREGNANCY

Do you have problems with your teeth or jaw?

Do you brush and floss your teeth regularly?

When was the last time you saw your dentist?

If you have tooth decay, sore or bleeding gums, or have not seen your dentist in the last 6 to 12 months, make a dental appointment. It is safe and important to visit a dentist during your pregnancy.

HELPFUL TIPS TO CONTROL NAUSEA AND VOMITING

- [ ] *Get up slowly.*
- [ ] *When you first wake up, eat a few crackers or some dry toast, and then rest for 15 minutes.*
- [ ] *Drink small amounts of fluids often during the day. Avoid drinking fluids during meals.*
- [ ] *Eat smaller amounts of food and eat often. Do not skip meals.*
- [ ] *Sniff fresh lemons, drink lemonade, or eat slices of watermelon.*
- [ ] *Try salty, dry foods such as crackers.*

(Continued)

women in Canada (about 4,000 women per year) suffer from severe nausea and vomiting. The lack of food, fluids, and nutrients may be harmful to their health and the well-being of their baby.

If it is not treated, severe nausea and vomiting can cause a woman to lose weight and can create an electrolyte imbalance. Electrolytes—such as sodium, calcium, chloride, magnesium, and phosphate—play an important role in making sure that the body works normally. When electrolytes are not in proper balance, this can cause health problems for pregnant women and their babies. It's important to talk to your health care provider if you have nausea and vomiting during pregnancy.

Acupressure and acupuncture treatments

These treatments have helped many pregnant women control their nausea and vomiting. About 30% of women find that the treatments relieve their symptoms. A person trained in this system will stimulate a certain point on your forearm. Bracelets used for seasickness (Sea-Band) also work on the same acupressure point.

Taking medicines or herbal products to control nausea and vomiting

It is always important talk to your health care provider before taking any medicines or herbal products during pregnancy, but for nausea and vomiting there are a couple that you can safely try. Ginger has been found to help many women. Very pure sources of ginger are available over-the-counter, formulated for nausea.

Vitamin B6 (pyridoxine) has also been found by many to be helpful for nausea and is something you can try, along with some of the tips listed in the sidebar.

It is best to speak to your health care provider if these solutions do not give you relief.

To learn more about surviving morning sickness and taking medications and herbal products when you are pregnant, visit the Motherisk Program's website at www.motherisk.org.

Prescription medications

Diclectin is the only prescription medication approved by Health Canada for the treatment of nausea and vomiting in pregnancy. It has been extensively tested and proven to be safe for mothers and babies and is effective. For very severe nausea and vomiting, there are other medications that your doctor may prescribe. If none of the suggestions have helped, your health care provider will recommend other measures.

Tender, painful breasts

You may want to get a good support bra and wear it all the time, even at night. Make sure it fits properly and that it has full, rounded cups with wide shoulder straps.

Feeling tired

During the first few months of pregnancy, you may feel very tired. It is normal to feel this way. Many things are happening inside your body. Your metabolism has increased, which takes a lot of your energy. Also, one of the pregnancy hormones (progesterone) makes women feel sleepy.

The best advice is to not try to fight the way you feel. Pay attention to your body, and when you need to rest or take a nap, just do it! Many women who never nap find themselves needing a little daytime rest. If you work outside the home, find a quiet place to relax and close your eyes when you have breaks. If this is impossible, lie down as soon as you get home from work.

STOP CHANGING THE CAT'S LITTER BOX

Parasites are all around us. Most will not harm us or our unborn children. Toxoplasmosis can harm your unborn baby. This disease is caused by a tiny parasite that lives in one animal and is passed on to other animals through its bowel movements (feces). Although it is rare for an adult to have any symptoms when he or she comes in contact with the parasite, there is a small risk of birth defects if a woman is exposed to the parasite during her pregnancy.

To be safe, avoid eating under-cooked meat, chicken, or wild game when you are pregnant. Wear rubber gloves when you handle raw meat or chicken. If you have a cat, ask someone else to change the litter box. If you must do the job yourself, follow these steps:

- *Wear gloves.*
- *Do not inhale the dust from the litter box.*
- *Wash your hands well when you have finished.*

Also, avoid digging in a garden or lawn where cats may have had bowel movements.

Varicose veins

Pregnancy increases the amount of blood in your body. This change supports the growing fetus, but it can result in enlarged veins in your legs. Varicose veins may surface for the first time or worsen during late pregnancy, when your uterus puts greater pressure on the veins in your legs. Changes in your hormones during pregnancy also may play a role. Varicose veins generally improve shortly after the baby is born. To help, rest and put up your feet as often as you can. Move around if you stand for long periods. Ask your health care provider about special support stockings.

Headaches

Headaches are quite common during pregnancy. In most cases, there is no reason for alarm. If you have headaches all the time or if they are very severe (blurred vision, nausea, or spots appear in front of your eyes), contact your health care provider.

If you have a headache, the following suggestions may help:

- Lie down in a dark, cool room.
- Place a cool cloth on your forehead.
- Try back stretches or, if available, have someone give you a neck massage.
- Try to eat small meals often. Sometimes, the headache is linked to low blood sugar, especially if you have a feeling of nausea and do not feel like eating.
- Talk to your health care provider before taking pain medication for a headache.

The need to urinate often

Do you need to go to the bathroom more often? This is normal during early pregnancy for these reasons:

- Your growing uterus is pressing on your bladder.
- Your kidneys are making more urine.

Even though your bladder feels full, you may pass only a little urine. Also, the pressure may cause urine to leak out when you move or cough. Kegel exercises may help (see page 59). If you feel any pain when you urinate, you may have an infection, and you should talk to your health care provider.

Light bleeding or spotting

Many women have a small amount of harmless spotting early in their pregnancy. They go on to give birth to healthy babies. If you have any bleeding at all, take it seriously and contact your health care provider. If the bleeding persists and is heavier than a period—especially if you have cramps—you may be at risk of a miscarriage. Seek emergency treatment.

Fainting

Feeling faint is common during pregnancy. It may be caused by:

- Higher hormone levels
- Changes to your circulation system
- Low blood sugar levels

If you feel light-headed, try eating a small nutritious snack between meals. When you feel faint, sit down and put your head between your knees. Loosen any tight clothing and place a cool, wet cloth on your forehead or on the back of your neck. If the feeling does not go away, contact your health care provider.

PROTECT YOUR UNBORN CHILD

The best way to protect an unborn child in a car crash is to protect the mother. Pregnant women should always wear the lap and shoulder seat belts.

- *The straps should be placed carefully above and below your stomach.*

- *The lap belt should be snug and low over the pelvic bones and not pressing against the soft stomach area.*

- *The shoulder belt should be worn across the chest.*

When worn the correct way, the seat belt will not harm the baby.

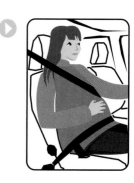

Diabetes

An increasing number of Canadians are developing diabetes, and this includes many women who will become pregnant. There are two most common types of diabetes—type 1 and type 2—and a third type called *gestational diabetes* that can develop later in pregnancy (see Chapter Three). Diabetes is when the body does not produce or properly use insulin. Insulin is a hormone that tells the cells how to convert sugars and starches into energy.

Types of Diabetes	
Type 1	*Type 2*
When the pancreas fails to produce any insulin at all	*When the pancreas fails to produce enough insulin or when the body cannot use this insulin properly*
↓	↓
A person with type 1 diabetes must inject insulin to allow glucose (sugars from food) to enter and fuel the cells of the body.	*A person with type 2 diabetes may be able to control his or her blood sugars (glucose levels) by eating properly and by getting enough regular exercise to burn off extra glucose.*

If you have diabetes

During pregnancy women with type 1 diabetes must test their blood glucose (blood sugar) levels every day and then inject the right amount of insulin to keep those levels normal. For some people, good control of their blood glucose levels is not easy. When a woman who must use insulin becomes pregnant, this challenge becomes even greater. If you have type 1 diabetes you will need to be carefully followed through your pregnancy to help control your sugars. Depending on where you live, there may be a special team that works with you, including diabetes educators, nurses, and specialized physicians.

If you have diabetes that you control with your diet and exercise, you may be able to continue to control your sugars with attention to diet and exercise and carefully monitoring your blood glucose levels. As the demands of pregnancy increase, your management may need to be changed. If the sugars are not well controlled, you may be advised to use insulin throughout the pregnancy. Women who are taking metformin can safely continue taking it during the first phase of pregnancy, but your doctor will advise you how best to control your blood sugars.

Good control of blood glucose levels is very important for a healthy pregnancy, especially during the month when the baby is conceived and during the first trimester. Pregnant women with poorly controlled blood glucose levels are more likely to have a large baby, difficulties during birth, and a baby with birth defects. During your pregnancy, eating a healthy, balanced diet and exercising will help your own and your baby's health.

A woman with diabetes should be monitored by a health care team. This team should include someone who is a diabetes expert. As the pregnancy advances, the team will help control blood glucose levels.

If you have high blood pressure

If you have high blood pressure and did not see your doctor prior to becoming pregnant, it is important to see your doctor as soon as you can after becoming pregnant. Managing your blood pressure well is important for both you and your baby.

COULD IT BE DEPRESSION?

One woman in 10 suffers from depression during pregnancy. Check with your health care provider if you have any of the symptoms in the following list for at least 2 weeks or if you are worried about any one of these symptoms:

- [ ] *Depressed mood or extreme sadness*
- [ ] *Crying spells for no apparent reason*
- [ ] *Guilty thoughts or feelings of worthlessness or hopelessness*
- [ ] *Restlessness, lack of control, or lack of energy*
- [ ] *Difficulty concentrating or disorganized thoughts*
- [ ] *Feelings of guilt or inadequacy as a mother-to-be*
- [ ] *Changes in sleep or appetite (for example, sleeping or eating too little or too much)*
- [ ] *Withdrawing from your partner, family, friends, coworkers*

Your emotions during pregnancy

Taking care of your physical health is an important part of having a healthy pregnancy. You also need to take care of your mental health.

When you are pregnant, it is normal to have mood swings. One minute you can be feeling happy about being pregnant, and the next you might find yourself worried and stressed out about the health of your baby or what will happen once the baby is born. The hormones that support your pregnancy and your baby also affect your moods. Although some women may feel moody all the way through their pregnancy, the highs and lows are most common between the 6th and 10th weeks and then again in the third trimester when the body is getting ready for labour and birth.

Here are some tips to help you take care of your emotional health when you are pregnant:

- Stay active and eat well.
- Take time to relax and rest.
- Avoid stressful situations and people.
- Share your thoughts and feelings with someone you trust.

Relationship stresses

As much as pregnancy can be a happy and hopeful time, it can also be very stressful for you and your partner. Financial worries and worry about raising the baby are common for both partners. Talk to your health care professional about your concerns.

Coping with stress and finding support

Everyone has some stress in his or her life, but having too much stress is not healthy, especially during pregnancy. Stress during pregnancy has been linked to preterm birth and low birth weight in babies.

The amount of support you receive from the people around you can have a direct effect on how much stress you feel during your pregnancy. If you receive very little support, you may feel lonely and depressed.

Although pregnancy is a joyous time for most couples, the changes and adjustments can sometimes cause strain in your relationship and increase your stress level. If you are not in a relationship, you may be feeling stressed about being alone. Events you did not expect may happen even during pregnancy. This can also increase your stress levels.

If you find that your stress level is rising, look for community resources that can help you find ways to reduce your stress and deal with challenges.

Ways to reduce your stress

Women with too much stress can learn healthy ways to deal with it. Here are some tips:

Talk about it. Share the joys, problems, and worries of pregnancy with someone close to you. This can make your pregnancy seem less stressful. If, for some reason, you do not have the support of your partner, try to spend time with other people whose company you enjoy.

Learn about pregnancy and childbirth. Attend prenatal classes and meet other pregnant women. The breathing and concentration exercises you will learn for childbirth can help you relax now. By knowing what to expect and being prepared, you can reduce any worry you may be feeling about the birth itself. Working with your health care provider and support person to prepare a birth plan may help, too. (Read about birth plans on page 116.)

Get active. Exercise can lift your spirits and reduce stress.

Rest and relax. Make sure you are sleeping enough. Learn other ways to rest and relax. Your public library may have books and audiotapes about reducing stress and learning to relax.

Abuse during pregnancy

The most common forms of abuse are verbal, emotional, or psychological. Pregnancy can be a very stressful time for both partners, and with stress comes an increased risk of abusive behavior. It is not healthy for either partner to be in an abusive situation, but it is particularly harmful for the pregnant woman.

One in 12 women in Canada is a victim of physical violence. Physical abuse during pregnancy can hurt both the mother and her unborn baby. It may even cause the baby to be born too early or too small. Some unborn babies have died because of abuse suffered by their mothers.

If you are pregnant and are a victim of any form of abuse, you probably feel very alone. You need help **now.**

No one deserves to be abused. Sometimes, abuse in a family can leave a woman feeling ashamed. She may feel that the abuse is her fault. Please ask for help. Talk to your health care provider. He or she will support you and help you find the community resources you need.

If you would like to learn more about abuse and places you can call or visit for help, visit www.sheltersafe.ca. Read more about family violence at www.phac-aspc.gc.ca/sfv-avf/index-eng.php or call the Assaulted Women's Helpline at 1-866-863-0511.

ARE YOU IN AN ABUSIVE RELATIONSHIP?

☐ *Do disagreements end by fighting?*

☐ *Do you feel frightened by what your partner says or does?*

☐ *Have you ever been hit, pushed, shoved, or slapped by your partner?*

☐ *Is your partner mean to you or does he or she make you feel worthless or stupid?*

☐ *Have you ever been forced to have sex against your will?*

If you have answered yes to any of these questions, discuss this with your health care provider or someone who can help.

▶ WHEN THE ONE WHO LOVES YOU HURTS YOU

CYCLE OF VIOLENCE

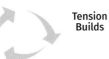

I'm Sorry
Romance
Stage

Tension
Builds

Explosive Event

Types of abuse

There are many different kinds of abuse. They all harm a pregnant woman and her growing baby in some way. If you live with abuse, always remember that it is not your fault and you can get help. Talk to your health care provider if you are living with any of these kinds of abuse.

Types of abuse	
Physical abuse	• Pushing, shoving, hitting, slapping, or kicking • Destroying personal property • Limiting mobility by tying you down or locking you in a room • Using a weapon or other objects to threaten or hurt • Denying access to a health care provider, such as a doctor, midwife, or dentist • Taking away assistive devices for a disability, such as a guide dog or a cane
Psychological or emotional abuse	• Threatening to take the children away (threatening to leave with the children or make a report to child protective services) • Stalking or harassing behaviour • Controlling how you spend your time • Isolating you from family and friends • Threatening to hurt a person or an animal you care for
Verbal abuse	• Name-calling or other verbal means of attacking self-esteem • Humiliating you in the presence of others • Giving you the silent treatment
Sexual abuse	• Denying sexual activity or forcing you into unwanted sexual acts • Forcing you to continue a pregnancy or to have an abortion • Infecting you with a sexually transmitted infection Note: Even if someone is married or engaged, a partner cannot force you to have sex.

Spiritual abuse	• Belittling your spiritual beliefs
	• Not allowing you to attend the place of worship of your choice
	• Forcing participation in religious activities or organizations
Financial abuse	• Limiting access to family finances
	• Spending the family money
Digital abuse	• Verbal or psychological or emotional abuse perpetrated online
	• Internet stalking
	• E-mailing inappropriate pictures and texts
	• Constant texting as surveillance
	• Phone tracking

Source: Best Start, Abuse in Pregnancy: Information and Strategies for Prenatal Education.

Miscarriages do happen

One of the most stressful and disappointing things that can happen in a pregnancy is a miscarriage. They occur in 15% to 20% of pregnancies, and they happen most often during the first 8 weeks. Some miscarriages take place before a woman misses a menstrual cycle or is even aware that she is pregnant.

The cause of miscarriage is often unknown. It may be the body's natural response to an embryo that is not growing properly and would not be able to survive. Although the 15% to 20% rate for miscarriages seems to be high, it includes those that happen in the very early days of a pregnancy.

It's important for all pregnant women to take any vaginal bleeding seriously. You should also know that 20% of mothers have some bleeding before the 20th week and that about half of these pregnancies will continue without further problems.

Bleeding does not always mean a miscarriage, but you should let your health care provider know if you are experiencing any bleeding. You should seek urgent medical attention if the bleeding soaks a thick sanitary pad every hour, over a period of 2 hours. Any bleeding should be reported to your health care provider.

Although a miscarriage does not affect most women's future fertility or their ability to carry a child to full term, wait at least one regular menstrual cycle before trying to become pregnant again. Also, emotional healing is just as important as physical healing. Any woman who has a miscarriage should expect to feel a range of emotions as well as physical discomforts. Grieving enables the woman to begin the healing process, which is unique for each person. Talk to your health care provider about support available for you. Pregnancy and Infant Loss Network (PAIL) also has a good support network: www.pailnetwork.ca.

MY DUE DATE:

Date:

Week of pregnancy:

Blood pressure:

Weight:

My pregnancy journal
First trimester

This visit takes place about 4 weeks after your first appointment. In most cases, you will not have a complete physical exam. You should expect to be weighed and have your blood pressure taken. Your health care provider will check the growth of your uterus and may also check your baby's heart rate.

At this visit, you and your health care provider will discuss the results of any tests. You may also talk about any other testing or actions that may be recommended.

As with every prenatal visit, be prepared to tell your health care provider about any concerns or questions you may have. Filling out this section of the handbook can help you prepare for each visit. Bring this handbook with you and take notes during your appointment.

If possible, it's a good idea for your partner or support person (close friend, mother, or other family member) to attend a visit to your health care provider at least once. This will give him or her a chance to meet the person who is caring for you and voice any concerns or questions he or she may have.

THINGS TO DISCUSS WITH MY
HEALTH CARE PROVIDER

- What are the benefits and risks of genetic testing?

- What advice do you have to help me control nausea and vomiting?

- How much weight should I gain?

- Am I eating the right foods?

- Is it okay to have sex?

- Am I doing too much or too little exercise?

- I have concerns about abuse in my relationship.

- How do I know I am doing Kegel exercises correctly?

- Other concerns:

My to-do list

My test results

Hemoglobin (normal 110–120 mg/L):

Blood type:

Immunity to rubella: Yes/No

Immunity to chicken pox: Yes/No

Other results:

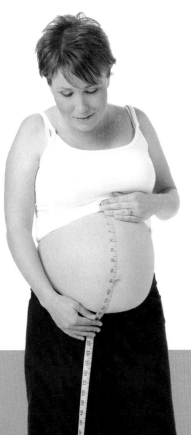

CHAPTER THREE

Gentle growth:
the second trimester

MEASURING YOUR BABY'S GROWTH

A routine part of your prenatal check-up is a measurement called symphysis-fundal height (SFH). Your health care provider will measure your abdomen to see how well your baby is growing.

The SFH is the distance from your pubic bone to the top of your uterus—this part of the uterus is called the fundus. The fundus usually reaches to the top of the pubic bone by about the 12th week of pregnancy. It reaches under your rib cage by the 36th week. Between the 18th and 30th weeks, the height of the fundus (in centimetres) is close to the age of the baby in weeks.

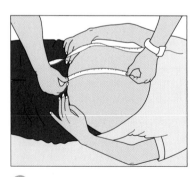

▶ *Measuring your baby's growth*

You have now reached the second trimester. This trimester will last from the 13th to the 26th week. You will begin to feel more like you did before pregnancy began. Morning sickness and minor discomforts are likely behind you.

You may feel some new discomforts, but many women enjoy this part of their pregnancy because their bodies are adapting to the pregnancy and their babies are making themselves known. It is a time of gentle growth.

Your baby will be growing quickly and will soon be big enough for you to feel the rolls, somersaults, and kicks. Babies like to exercise.

In this chapter, we will talk about the following:

- Preterm labour and birth
- Work
- Swelling
- Backaches

We will also provide places for you to keep track of new information about you and your baby.

Your changing body

During your second trimester, you may feel calmer and more settled. The placenta is where the baby's umbilical cord attaches to your uterus, bringing oxygen and nutrients from the mother's circulation to the baby's. The placenta is an amazing organ. It now takes on one of its unique roles: producing the hormones that sustain your pregnancy. (See page 4 to learn more about the placenta.)

You will also notice that your body's shape and size will begin to change. Everyone looks different in her pregnancy. Your friends or family may say that you seem "small" or look "large." If you have been having regular prenatal visits, you will know that your baby is growing just fine.

So what determines your size during pregnancy? Your height, weight, and build—before you were pregnant—and whether or not this is your first pregnancy will have an impact on how your body grows and changes. Short women tend to look bigger. Large-boned or taller women tend to look smaller. Some women carry smaller babies because of their ethnic background. Second-time mothers tend to have bigger bellies because the muscles of the abdomen and uterus were stretched before.

The colour of your skin (pigmentation) may be changing because of shifting hormones. You may develop a brownish, vertical line down the middle of your belly. This is called the ***linea nigra***. Some women develop brownish, uneven marks around their eyes and over their nose and cheeks. These marks usually go away when hormone levels return to normal after your baby's birth.

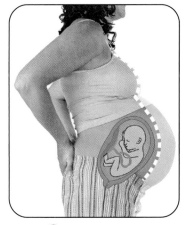

 Second trimester

As your breasts begin to get ready to feed your baby, you may notice a little **colostrum** leaking from the nipples. Colostrum is the first breast milk your body produces. It is a yellow fluid that contains antibodies to protect your baby against infections.

As a way to get ready for birth, hormones in your body will soften the ligaments and cartilage in your pelvis and back.

Your growing baby

At about the 16th to 18th week, the recommended ultrasound will show that your fetus is really looking like a baby—nicely formed with all body systems in place, working well, and beginning to mature. If you could see the skin it would look red because the blood vessels are close to the surface—but you won't be able to see that on an ultrasound! If you could, you would also see that a layer of fat is starting to form under the skin, and a thick coating of a white, waxy-like substance called **vernix** may be present on the surface of the body. Between 18 and 24 weeks the fetus will also begin to suck and swallow amniotic fluid.

The eyelids open and close by 26 weeks. The fingernails are full length and many babies have a visible hairline. Eyebrows and scalp hair become visible at the end of the 20th week and by 24 weeks you can even see the eyelashes. The amniotic sac is filled with a large amount of fluid that contains nutrients for growth and small amounts of the baby's urine. The umbilical cord is thick, strong, and very firm, which helps prevent knots from forming.

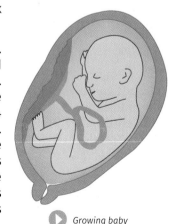

▶ *Growing baby*

About fetal movement

Babies move their arms and legs to exercise and to find a more comfortable position. If you are pregnant for the first time, you may not feel your baby move until about your 19th week. If this is not your first pregnancy, you may begin to feel movement sooner, at around the 17th week. From that point on, you should feel your baby move at different times of the day, every day. Keep in mind that babies sleep at certain times of the day and will be more active at other times. You may be asked to keep track of your baby's movements by counting the number of kicks you feel. (See page 111 for how to count movements.)

Weight gain during the second trimester

Remember to review the guide and how much weight to gain and what to eat discussed in Chapter Two. At this stage in pregnancy, you may need to eat a little more to get the right nutrition for you and your baby. Two to three extra servings or healthy snacks should be enough for most women, but if you are underweight or overweight, you may need some specific advice to help adjust your diet.

About work

In most normal pregnancies, the type of work you do is not usually a problem. However, strenuous work or standing up for a long time has been linked to problems such as small babies, preterm labour, and miscarriage. To find out if your work is too demanding for a pregnant woman, answer the questions in the sidebar on page 101.

You may be at risk if you work with certain chemicals. Governments have set rules to limit exposure to toxic chemicals. To find out more about environmental hazards and pregnancy, see the Motherisk website at www.motherisk.org and check government health and safety regulations.

Common discomforts during the second trimester

Backaches

Your growing belly will make you lean back to find your centre of gravity, which then strains your back muscles. The weight of the uterus in your pelvis, combined with joint movement and joint softening, can also give you backaches during pregnancy. To prevent backaches, try the following:

- Always try to sit up straight.
- Avoid wearing high heels.
- Avoid standing for long periods of time.

Your health care provider may suggest that you see a licensed massage therapist, physiotherapist, or chiropractor. Yoga, stretching, and learning new ways to relax may help, too. Read about pelvic tilt exercises on page 59. Be sure to change your body position often and take time to lie down, put your feet up, and relax. Try using heat, ice packs, or massages to ease the pain.

Constipation

During pregnancy, your food tends to move slowly through your bowels. This slowing down can lead to *constipation* (irregular or difficult bowel movements). If you are taking iron supplements, they can cause constipation (and may turn your stools black). To help keep the stool (bodily waste) from becoming dry and hard, drink at least eight glasses of fluid (water, milk, or juice) daily. Getting regular exercise and eating a healthy, balanced diet with plenty of fibre will help, too. Foods that are high in fibre include:

- Vegetables
- Fruit
- Grain products made of whole grains
- Legumes such as beans, peas and lentils
- Nuts and seeds

Visit www.dietitians.ca/Downloads/Factsheets/Food-Sources-of-Soluble-Fibre.aspx for the soluble fibre content from a variety of foods. If needed, your health care provider may suggest a bulk-forming agent or stool softener.

Feeling dizzy when you are flat on your back

Lying on your back can sometimes make you feel light-headed and dizzy. Find a position—lying on your side or on an incline—that makes you comfortable. Anything that makes you comfortable and lets you get some rest is fine.

Groin pain

The round ligament that holds the uterus in place sometimes goes into spasms when it stretches as your baby grows. This stretching may feel like a stabbing pain on one or both sides of your lower belly, or it can feel like a dull ache. These pains seem to be most common in the second trimester. It may help to avoid turning your waist quickly. When you do feel pain, lean into it (bend toward the pain) to help relax the tension on the muscles. Lie down and get some rest. Groin pain may feel similar to preterm labour. If the pain continues or gets worse—and if it does not go away when you

---

HELP FOR INDIGESTION AND HEARTBURN

THINGS YOU CAN DO

- *Avoid lying down for 1 to 2 hours after eating.*
- *Raise the head of your bed (30 degrees or 6 inches).*
- *Wear loose clothing, especially around the waist.*
- *Avoid exercise after eating.*
- *Eat smaller amounts of food more often.*
- *Eat slowly and chew your food well.*
- *Drink fluids between meals rather than during meals.*

FOODS YOU MIGHT WANT TO AVOID

Not everyone finds the same foods troublesome, but here is a list of foods that many people find make heartburn worse:

- *Fatty or deep-fried foods*
- *Rich desserts, such as cheesecake*
- *Spicy foods*

(Continued)

HELP FOR INDIGESTION
AND HEARTBURN (CONTINUED)

- *Onions and garlic*
- *Citrus fruit, such as oranges, grapefruit, and lemons*
- *Tomatoes*
- *Spearmint and peppermint*
- *Coffee and tea*
- *Chocolate*
- *Carbonated beverages (soda pop, drinks with bubbles)*

change positions—go to the obstetrics ward of your hospital or visit your health care provider.

Hemorrhoids

Many expectant mothers will develop *hemorrhoids* (swollen veins in the rectum). Hemorrhoids often flare up during pregnancy because the growing uterus places a lot of pressure on these veins. If a woman strains to have a bowel movement because she has hard stools, the hemorrhoids become worse and may push out around the anal opening. Sometimes they are painful and bleed. Try to eat foods that will reduce constipation (see "Constipation" on pages 92 to 93). Your health care provider may suggest ointments to help shrink the hemorrhoids, or you can try cool witch hazel compresses.

Indigestion and heartburn

If you have a burning feeling at the back of your throat, lower in your food pipe (esophagus), or in your stomach, you may be suffering from indigestion. This is often caused by pregnancy hormones and the pressure of your growing uterus against your stomach.

Things that may help include the following:

- Eating small amounts of food more often
- Eating slowly
- Chewing your food well
- Drinking fluids between rather than during meals
- Avoiding caffeine and greasy, spicy foods that cause gas
- Sitting upright after a meal to give the food time to pass from the stomach into the intestine
- Wearing loose clothing

Talk to your health care provider before taking any antacids. Antacids can cause a negative effect, in which your stomach produces even more acids after the antacid wears off. As well, antacids that contain aluminum may make it hard to absorb certain minerals from food.

Dry or itchy skin

Avoid using harsh soaps because they tend to wash away the natural oils in your skin. Instead, use a mild soap with fewer added ingredients. Avoid lying in a tub of water for too long; this can also dry out your skin. Putting oil or an oatmeal-based softener in the bath will help. After a bath or shower, apply body lotion to your damp skin. This will help keep your skin softer.

Stretch marks

Many women get stretch marks—reddish streaks—on their breasts, belly, and thighs during pregnancy. Many women rub oils (such as vitamin E oil or lanolin) on their bellies. This may not affect the stretch marks, but it is not harmful and can be relaxing.

Swelling of your legs, ankles, and feet

A small amount of swelling in your legs, ankles, and feet is normal during pregnancy. This type of swelling builds up each day and should mostly disappear by the time you get up the next morning. It can be more of a problem if the weather is quite warm. Make sure you drink plenty of fluids (eight glasses a day) and do not remove salt from your diet. Your body needs some salt for day-to-day functions. If your hands or face swell, it may mean that you have a more serious problem, such as high blood pressure (see page 112).

TIPS TO HELP REDUCE THE SWELLING IN YOUR LEGS, ANKLES, AND FEET

- *Get regular exercise using your legs (e.g., swimming, walking, etc.).*

- *Do not cross your legs when you are seated.*

- *Wear support hose and avoid socks with tight bands of elastic around the top.*

- *Do not stand for too long.*

- *Raise your legs above the level of your heart as often as you can.*

- *Drink eight glasses of fluids (preferably water or milk) each day. How much you need to drink can depend on many factors, such as your activity level. At least eight glasses a day would be a good beginning. If your urine is yellow (one sign of dehydration), increase your fluid intake. Your urine should be pale in colour.*

- *Do not remove salt from your diet.*

When there are complications in the second trimester

Abdominal surgery

Sometimes abdominal surgery is needed when a woman is pregnant (for example, for appendicitis). If you need to have surgery, your care will be coordinated between the surgical and obstetric services in your hospital. Surgery that is wanted but not essential (that is, elective) should be avoided until after the baby is born.

Accidents

It is true that we are more accident-prone in pregnancy—research has proven it! Knowing that, it is a good idea to take a few precautions to prevent accidents. Wear well-fitting shoes, use bannisters on staircases, watch for tripping hazards (especially as your belly begins to expand and your feet disappear from view)! Be more vigilant when you are tired, use night lights if you get up at night, and try to avoid distractions in the kitchen.

But if you are in an accident, especially a fall or a car accident, be sure to contact your health care provider. In most cases you will be asked to come to the hospital for you and your baby to be checked over.

Bleeding

A small amount of bleeding can happen if the placenta starts to pull away from the lining of the uterus. Always contact your health care provider if you notice any bleeding, even if you have been treated for bleeding before.

Placenta previa

When the placenta implants and grows over the opening of the cervix (the bottom of the uterus) it is called *placenta previa*. It can cause heavy bleeding during labour. In most cases, the condition is found during routine ultrasound testing. Bed rest for the last few weeks of pregnancy and caesarean birth before labour begins are the usual recommendations.

Diabetes in pregnancy

For women who had diabetes before pregnancy, the care that started in the first trimester will be continuing throughout pregnancy, with close monitoring of both mother and baby.

For some women, pregnancy hormones change the way their bodies use insulin. They may develop a type of diabetes that only happens during pregnancy called ***gestational diabetes.*** Your health care provider may recommend a test for gestational diabetes at around 24 to 28 weeks.

Most pregnant women with gestational diabetes will be able to control their blood sugar levels by following a special diet and exercising. A small number may require insulin injections or pills to control their blood sugar levels. With knowledge, good control, and professional care by a health care team, most women with gestational diabetes have a safe pregnancy and a healthy baby.

For most, the condition goes away after the baby is born. Some women may develop diabetes or be at risk for heart disease later in life, so it is important to continue to follow a healthy diet and lifestyle after pregnancy.

For information about the special needs of women who have type 1, or insulin-dependent, diabetes before they become pregnant, see pages 76 to 77.

Fibroids

Large fibroids—growths in the muscle wall of the uterus—can push the uterus out of its natural shape and can cause pain and preterm labour. If the fibroids grow large enough to deform the uterus and are found before you become pregnant, they may be removed. Small fibroids usually don't cause problems during pregnancy.

Hypertension (hypertensive disorders of pregnancy)

High blood pressure in pregnancy begins to show up in the second trimester. You will have your blood pressure checked at every visit. The most important difference is made by an early diagnosis. Hypertensive disorders require careful management and will be treated in different ways, depending on how serious it is. (Read more about it in "High blood pressure during pregnancy" on page 112.)

Infections

Infections of the vagina, cervix, kidney, and bladder are common during pregnancy and must be treated. The signs of an infection in your vagina or cervix include unusual discharge from your vagina, pain in your pelvis or groin area, or a fever. If you suspect an infection, contact your health care provider.

Bladder infections

Bladder infections sometimes can be hard to detect. The common signs of an infection in your bladder are as follows:

- Pain when you urinate
- Having to urinate more often than usual
- Only passing urine in very small amounts—even though you feel like your bladder is full

This kind of infection can be treated easily with antibiotics. Your health care provider will recommend antibiotics that are safe for you and your baby.

An upper urinary tract infection (which involves the kidneys) is more serious. It can cause chills, fever, nausea, vomiting, backache, pain in the side of your body, and pain in your lower abdomen.

Women who are prone to bladder infections should be very careful when they are pregnant. These infections can lead to preterm labour.

Preterm labour

Preterm labour means that your labour begins before 37 weeks of pregnancy—weeks before the baby is supposed to be born.

Preterm babies are more fragile, and preterm labour is one of the most common problems in pregnancy. It causes 75% of all deaths in otherwise healthy newborns. Being born early can cause the baby to have lifelong challenges. In general, the earlier a baby is born, the more severe the problems. Babies born before the 25th week are at high risk of not surviving or of having significant health problems.

It's important to know the early signs of preterm labour because sometimes it can be stopped or delayed. The sooner you notice preterm labour, the more time there is to give medicine that can help the baby and to treat any of the conditions that might be causing preterm labour.

What causes preterm labour?

We do not know what causes preterm labour. About half of all preterm labours begin for no obvious reason in women who seem to be having a normal pregnancy. Certain things seem associated with a woman's chances of going into early labour (see sidebar "Are you at risk for preterm labour?").

ARE YOU AT RISK FOR PRETERM LABOUR?

As you read this list, check off any statements that apply to you.

☐ *I do not have regular prenatal care.*

☐ *I have high blood pressure.*

☐ *There is a lot of stress in my life.*

☐ *My partner or someone else abuses me in a physical or emotional way.*

☐ *I am pregnant with more than one fetus.*

☐ *A previous baby of mine was born too early.*

☐ *I weigh less than 45.5 kg (100 lbs).*

☐ *I have a chronic illness.*

☐ *I smoke.*

☐ *I quit smoking cigarettes, but not until after my 32nd week of pregnancy.*

☐ *I use recreational drugs.*

☐ *I have had a procedure on my cervix for an abnormal pap test.*

☐ *I work long hours (more than 8 hours a day) or do shift work.*

☐ *My work is physically demanding (strenuous).*

If you checked off one or more boxes, you are at risk for preterm labour. You should talk to your health care provider to learn how to help prevent preterm labour.

SIGNS OF PRETERM LABOUR AND OTHER SIGNS OF DISTRESS

Preterm labour can happen to anyone. There are ways to reduce the risk. Here are some signs of preterm labour:

- *Regular contractions of the uterus before your baby is due*
- *Low dull backache*
- *A feeling of pressure in the lower abdomen, the pelvis, or the lower back*

Learn the signs. Act right away, and find a way to go to the nearest hospital safely if you experience any of these:

- *Bleeding*
- *Leaking or a gush of fluid from your vagina*
- *Pain in your abdomen that you cannot explain*
- *A decrease in your baby's movement*
- *Unusual and constant headaches*
- *Blurred vision or spots before your eyes*
- *Feeling dizzy*
- *Dull pain in your lower back that does not go away*
- *Being in a motor vehicle accident*

As you've been reading this handbook, you have learned that the best way to have a healthy pregnancy and baby is to avoid risks and take care of your health.

Some interesting facts: The rate of premature births drops when women know the risks and signs of preterm labour and when women are involved and contribute to their own pregnancy record.

Some risk factors for preterm labour and tips on how you can reduce your risk

Smoking

It is best to quit smoking before or early in pregnancy. Quitting smoking is a healthy choice for you and your baby.

Talk to your health care provider about quitting. There are groups, helplines, online support, and one-on-one services to help women quit smoking. The use of nicotine replacement therapy products can be helpful, especially when using appropriate doses. Your health care provider can assist.

Street drugs

Taking recreational or street drugs during your pregnancy or while breastfeeding is harmful to you and your baby. Ask for help if you want to quit using recreational or street drugs.

Working too hard

Most women are able to work through their pregnancy, but some jobs are too strenuous and can increase your risk of a preterm birth. Learn about work that is too much for a pregnant woman (see sidebar "Is my work too physically demanding?" on page 101). Plan ahead to make sure you get time to rest every day. Do not feel guilty about resting. It is very important during pregnancy.

Physical and emotional abuse

When someone hurts you, they can also hurt your unborn baby. Even emotional abuse can lead to a preterm birth by raising your stress hormone levels. If you are being abused by your partner or someone else, seek help by calling a family crisis centre in your area. (Read the section "Abuse during pregnancy" on page 80.)

A weak cervix (incompetent cervix or cervical insufficiency)

This is a condition in which the cervix opens (dilates) too soon. The cervix is supposed to open when the baby is ready to be born, but in rare situations, the cervix can open too soon and cause premature birth. The pregnant woman may be unaware of the condition, but it can be discovered during a vaginal exam or when the size of the cervix is measured during an ultrasound. Sometimes, the problem can be treated by sewing the cervix closed and removing the stitch when the baby is full-term.

What you can do to prevent preterm labour

There are other things that you can do in an effort to try to prevent your baby from being born too soon.

- Visit your health care provider regularly during pregnancy.
- Eat a healthy diet.
- If you are being abused, call your local women's shelter and ask where you can go for help.
- Get plenty of rest.
- Learn ways to reduce stress.
- Avoid strenuous work.
- Avoid overexertion when exercising.
- Learn to recognize the signs of premature labour.
- Talk to your health care provider about what you should do if you are in preterm labour. Write down the phone numbers to call.

IS MY WORK TOO PHYSICALLY DEMANDING?

As you read this list, check off any statements that are true for you. When I am at work . . .

- ☐ *I stoop or bend over more than 10 times each hour.*
- ☐ *I climb a ladder more than three times during an 8-hour shift.*
- ☐ *I stand for more than 4 hours at one time.*
- ☐ *I climb stairs more than three times per shift.*
- ☐ *I work more than 40 hours per week.*
- ☐ *I work shift work.*
- ☐ *I will need to lift more than 23 kg (50 lbs) after the 20th week of my pregnancy.*
- ☐ *I will need to lift more than 11 kg (24 lbs) after 24 weeks.*
- ☐ *I will need to stoop, bend, or climb ladders after my 28th week.*
- ☐ *I will need to lift heavy items after my 30th week.*
- ☐ *I will need to stand still for more than 30 minutes of every hour after 32 weeks.*

If you checked off any of these boxes, parts of your work may not be right for you while you are pregnant. Your health care provider can help support your request for modified work at your workplace until after your baby is born. (Read more about work during pregnancy on pages 91 and 101.)

HOW TO FEEL AND COUNT CONTRACTIONS (TIGHTENINGS)

1. *Lie down.*
2. *Using your fingertips, gently feel the entire surface of your belly.*
3. *When you notice a contraction (a feeling of tightness or squeezing) time and record your contractions, from the start of the contraction to the start of the next contraction, as well as how long they last, for example, occur 10 minutes apart and last 30 seconds.*

WHEN SOMETHING GOES WRONG

- *Call the hospital and talk to a nurse in the birthing unit.*

  Phone number:

- *Call your health care provider.*

  Phone number:

Labour and checking for preterm labour

Labour begins when your uterus starts to tighten (contract) at regular intervals. The following will happen as labour begins and your body prepares for your baby's travel down the birth canal:

- The cervix will begin to thin out (efface) and open up (dilate).
- The mucous plug that formed during pregnancy to protect the entrance of your uterus may come loose. This will produce a bloody discharge called a "show."
- Your "water" may break—this is when the sac filled with amniotic fluid that surrounds your baby breaks.

The only way to know for sure if you are in preterm labour is to be checked by a health care provider. He or she will be able to tell if the contractions you are feeling are causing the cervix to open. An ultrasound might be done to learn more about the size and position of your baby as well as to measure the length of your cervix. When the cervix gets shorter, this is a sign that you could be in preterm labour. Many hospitals have a special test that involves checking for a substance in the vaginal fluid that shows whether a woman is in preterm labour or not.

If your contractions are thought to be real labour, and you are less than 37 weeks pregnant, then medications may be suggested to delay labour to help the baby's lungs and nervous system mature.

Preterm babies

Although only about 7 out of 100 babies are born preterm, they face more problems than other babies, and some may die. Normally, labour begins sometime after your 37th week of pregnancy and before the end of your 41st week. If labour starts before you reach your 37th week, your labour is called *preterm*.

Preterm babies can have problems because their body organs are not ready to work all by themselves—they are not mature enough. For example, a baby's lungs are not ready to function until close to the end of the pregnancy, so many preterm babies have breathing problems. Some preterm babies have severe problem with various organs and may have long-lasting complications.

Premature birth can also affect your baby's ability to do the following:

• Feed
• Fight infections
• See
• Hear
• Stay warm

If you are pregnant with more than one baby, you and your health care provider will work together to ensure that your babies are born as close to full-term as possible.

Preterm rupture of the membranes

When the sac of amniotic fluid breaks or leaks before your baby reaches full term, it is called *preterm rupture of the membranes*, or PROM. If your membranes rupture early, treatment depends on how much amniotic fluid is lost and how close to your due date you are. If this happens to you, contact your health care provider or go to the hospital right away.

MATERNITY AND PARENTAL LEAVES

Each province has different rules for maternity and parental leaves. For more information, see the Government of Canada Employment Insurance Maternity and Parental Benefits overview at www.esdc. gc.ca/en/ei/maternity_parental/ index.page.

Pregnant women may have access to government programs for maternity leave. If the need arises, and if required, your health care provider can advise you to stop work because of concerns about your health. Depending on your situation, you may still get paid while you are on leave.

Date:

Week of pregnancy:

Blood pressure:

Weight:

My pregnancy journal
Second trimester

As was the case with the last prenatal visit, your examination will include weighing and measuring you and your baby.

At 16 to 18 weeks, your health care provider may suggest a screening ultrasound test. The images from the ultrasound will let your health care provider check the baby's growth and well-being and help to confirm your baby's due date.

Don't forget to register for your prenatal classes.

**THINGS TO DISCUSS WITH MY
HEALTH CARE PROVIDER**

- *Am I at risk for preterm labour?*

- *Is my work too physically
  demanding?*

- *Who will be looking after my
  baby at the time of birth and for
  ongoing well-baby care?*

- *Other concerns:*

My to-do list

My test results:

Gestational diabetes test: (Normal = 3.8–7.8 mmol/L)

Ultrasound results:

Other results:

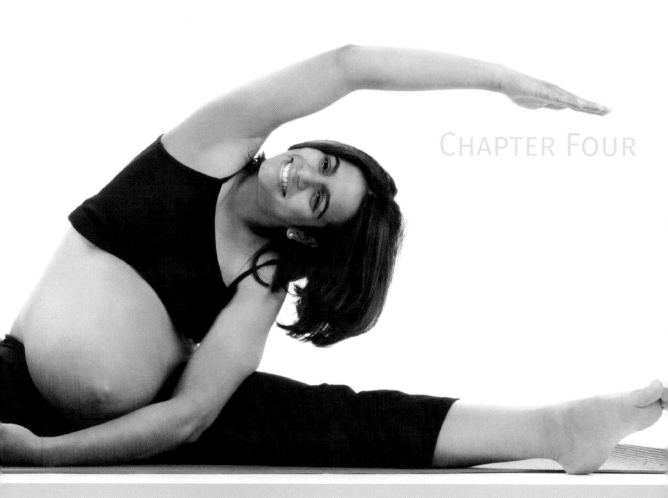

CHAPTER FOUR

The home stretch: the third trimester

Welcome to your third trimester! You are now looking forward to the arrival of your baby (and the end of your pregnancy).

So, let's look ahead to the rest of this handbook and how it will guide you through to the final stages of your pregnancy—and your baby's birth. In this chapter, we will talk about the following:

- Prenatal care during the third trimester
- Common concerns
- Things to consider when preparing a "birth plan" or birth preference list
- Introduction to breastfeeding

During your last month of pregnancy, your prenatal visits will be more frequent. You should expect to see your health care provider as often as once a week during the final month. Each visit will involve a check of your blood pressure, your urine, and the position of the baby. The goal will be to assess your general health and the health of your baby.

If you're wondering what to expect on the birth day, this chapter will provide information on some things that you need to plan well ahead for. There is advice on preparing a birth plan and on all the things that might go into yours, including a section on breastfeeding. How you will feed your baby is an important part of your plan.

Looking ahead, the next two chapters will cover the final 6 weeks before the day you give birth and then the birth itself. After that, the following chapter will discuss *you*—and getting back to "normal." Finally, we'll offer a chapter of information that will help get you started with your new family member.

Your changing body

During your third trimester, your pregnancy will become more visible. You will be amused by friends and even strangers who will look at your belly and tell you with confidence that you will be having a boy (if the belly pokes out) or a girl (more rounded profile). Overall those helpful friends do turn out to be right—about half the time.

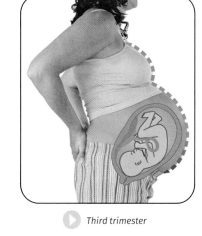

Third trimester

The top of your uterus will extend from above your navel to under your rib cage and your belly will stick out even further. This might make you feel more uncomfortable. You will feel pressure on your ribs and in your pelvis. Your abdominal muscles will feel stretched. You may feel sharp pains in your groin or vagina as your baby's head moves into your pelvis. As the baby moves lower into your pelvis, it will become easier to breathe and you may experience less indigestion.

In the next few weeks, you will be continuing to gain about a half a pound to a pound a week—depending on your starting weight. As you reach for those extra servings or snacks, continue to make them as healthy as possible, combining two or more food groups and eating at regular intervals.

LEG, CALF, AND FOOT CRAMPS

Many women feel cramps during the last 3 months of pregnancy, mostly at night. They are sudden cramps in the thighs, legs, calves, or feet. When you get a cramp, try this:

- *In spite of the pain, point your toes up or flex the foot toward your knee. This will help to stretch the muscle in the back of the calf.*

- *Keep your foot in this flexed position while you slowly and carefully make circles with your lower leg.*

- *Then, massage the cramped muscle to improve the blood supply to that part of your body.*

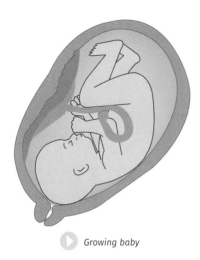

Growing baby

Your growing baby

Your baby was fully formed in the second trimester and will now keep growing in a steady way. At 25 to 26 weeks, the baby's weight will be between 700 and 900 grams (1.5 to 2 pounds). By 35 to 36 weeks, the baby will weigh 2,500 grams (5.5 pounds). By your due date, the weight will be between 3,000 and 4,000 grams (6.5 to 9 pounds).

Although all the organ systems are formed, they must still mature fully before they can function on their own. Between weeks 20 and 21, your baby's "breathing" movements become regular and between weeks 26 and 29, the baby would be able to breathe air if he or she were to be born. The baby's arms and legs are bent close to the body. The uterus is starting to feel crowded. You should still feel active movement each day, although the fetus (similar to a newborn) has active times and times of rest.

Baby continues to get ready to breastfeed. Rooting is usually seen around 32 weeks and the coordination of sucking, swallowing, and breathing occurs between 32 and 35 weeks.

Your prenatal care

Examinations will include measurements of your weight and blood pressure, urine tests, and your baby's position and growth. Toward the end of the third trimester, you may be offered vaginal exams to check if your cervix is changing in preparation for labour. This softening of the cervix means it is getting ready for birth.

You will be asked about your baby's movements. These details give your health care provider important information about your baby's health. You may also be asked to do daily movement counts.

Counting the baby's movements: Counting the kicks is an easy and reliable way to monitor your baby's well-being. By keeping track of fetal movements, you may reduce the risk of a stillbirth.

With a low-risk pregnancy, you may be advised to do fetal movement counts only if you notice decreased fetal movement in your third trimester.

With a high-risk pregnancy, your health care provider may advise that you should monitor fetal movements on a daily basis.

To count your baby's movements, take some quiet time in the evening while resting. If you are counting kicks and do not feel six movements within 2 hours, you should contact your health care provider.

Some facts about fetal movements:

- Most women feel regular movements after 24 weeks.
- The best time for counting may be in the evening, when there may be more fetal movement.
- Fetal movements may be better noticed when lying down.
- Smoking reduces fetal movements temporarily by reducing fetal blood flow.
- Some women do not feel fetal movements. An ultrasound scan may be helpful to observe the baby's movement.

Your health care provider may discuss other tests for your baby. Common tests that measure the well-being of a fetus are as follows:

Ultrasound: If there are any concerns about how your baby is growing, an ultrasound may be scheduled by your health care provider to monitor your baby's health by checking growth, movement, and the amount of amniotic fluid. The results of this test are often compared to any earlier ultrasounds.

Non-stress test: A non-stress test records your baby's heart rate. It may be done at your health care provider's clinic or at a hospital. The rate is measured for 20 to 30 minutes. If the baby is healthy, the test will show that the baby's heart rate rises with movement, just as yours does with exercise.

Stripping the membranes: Right near the time your baby is due to be born, your health care provider may suggest a procedure known as "stripping" the membranes.

Stripping the membranes is used to separate the amniotic sac membranes from the cervix, without breaking through the membranes. It can help your body get ready for the birth. It is a common practice that helps to prepare the cervix but is not necessary for all women. After explaining the risks and benefits and getting your consent, your health care provider will place a finger into your cervix (much like putting a finger into a small doughnut hole), and then circle the finger against the inside of the cervix to detach the membrane that is stuck to the sides. This procedure usually happens around your due date once the cervix has started to soften and open, and it can be performed in your health care provider's office. After it is done, most women have a bit of cramping that lasts a short time, along with a small amount of pink discharge.

When there are complications in the third trimester

High blood pressure during pregnancy

High blood pressure, also known as *hypertension,* is fairly common during pregnancy. Your health care provider will check your blood pressure often and may check for protein in your urine. You may also need to have some blood tests to see if your high blood pressure is a concern.

During pregnancy, a measurement of blood pressure greater than 140/90 or more is considered high, but your health care provider will also look at the difference between your blood pressure now and your blood pressure earlier in pregnancy. If it is much higher now, you may have hypertension, even if it is less than 140/90. Some women's blood pressure may be high before pregnancy and sometimes it becomes high during pregnancy.

There are some risk factors for pre-eclampsia: being pregnant with more than one baby, having had pre-eclampsia before, or having a medical condition such as hypertension or kidney disease (see the sidebar "Am I at risk for high blood pressure during pregnancy?" for other important risk factors). Pre-eclampsia can develop in any woman, and early diagnosis is important, so your blood pressure will be measured at every visit.

Pre-eclampsia can cause leaky blood vessels in the kidneys. This produces protein in the urine and high levels of swelling (read about normal swelling in "Swelling of your legs, ankles, and feet" on page 95). Extreme complications can include strokes, seizures, liver damage, and blood-clotting problems.

All types of high blood pressure are a concern for you and your baby. High blood pressure can cause poor growth and may even require giving birth early by inducing labour or a caesarean birth for the health of the mother or baby.

Treatment for high blood pressure in pregnancy

Some kinds of high blood pressure during pregnancy may be treated with rest. If you develop high blood pressure, you may be asked to stop work to allow more rest time at home. Your health

---

AM I AT RISK FOR HIGH BLOOD PRESSURE DURING PREGNANCY?

Check the boxes that apply to you:

☐ *This is my first pregnancy.*
☐ *I had high blood pressure before I got pregnant.*
☐ *I have diabetes.*
☐ *I have a medical condition that causes my kidneys not to work properly.*
☐ *I am carrying more than one baby.*
☐ *I am 40 years of age or older.*

If you checked any box, you are at an increased risk of developing hypertension in pregnancy.

About 5% to 10% of pregnant women develop a form of pregnancy-related high blood pressure or hypertension known as pre-eclampsia, or toxemia. When this happens, blood pressure is high and there may be protein detected in the urine. Symptoms include severe headaches, pain around your liver, irritability, swelling in the face, changes in vision, or seeing flashes of light.

- *You start labour before you reach 37 weeks.*
- *You reach full term, but your membranes rupture more than 18 hours before birth.*
- *You have an unexplained mild fever during labour.*
- *You have already had a baby who had a GBS infection.*
- *You have (or had) a bladder or kidney infection that was caused by the GBS bacteria.*

Signs of pre-eclampsia

If you have any of these symptoms, you could have a severe condition and should call your health care provider right away:

- *Pain in the upper right part of the belly*
- *Constant, severe, or changing headaches*
- *Spots in front of your eyes and/ or blurred vision*
- *Unusual swelling, particularly around the face*

care provider might also prescribe blood pressure medications to keep your blood pressure at a safe level for you and your baby.

Group B Streptococcus (GBS)

At about 36 weeks, you will likely be tested for group B Streptococcus (GBS) bacteria. This is different from strep throat. There is a small chance your baby could become infected by the GBS bacteria during childbirth. Babies with a GBS infection may have mild to severe problems that may affect their blood, brain, lungs, and spinal cord.

GBS bacteria are usually found in your vagina or rectum. They can infect your bladder, kidneys, or uterus. Infections from GBS are usually not serious for the pregnant woman, but they can be serious for the baby. They can be treated easily with antibiotics.

Testing for GBS

The most common way to test a woman for GBS bacteria is to obtain a sample from the vagina and rectum with a cotton swab. This is then placed in special liquid to see if the bacteria grow. Your health care provider may also test for bacteria in your urine.

Treatment for GBS

If at 36 weeks you test positive for GBS, you will not be treated right away because this has been found ineffective. Instead, you should be offered antibiotics during labour. If you have not been tested for GBS and fall into a high-risk group, then you may be treated with antibiotics during labour.

What to expect during labour and birth

Yes, it is a few weeks off, but it is important to be prepared. Birth is the most natural of natural processes, but most new mothers have had little to no experience with birth. Obstetrical health care in Canada has evolved to become a very family-centred experience, allowing women more choice in how their labour and birth will go forward, wherever they choose to give birth. Although the vast majority of women choose to give birth in hospitals, others choose birthing centres or home births when this option is available.

Efforts are made to ensure care is tailored to a woman's unique needs. That's why women are encouraged to prepare a birth plan that reflects their choices and desires.

Most hospitals and birth centres welcome family members, and this has been found to help the mother through the birth process and early postpartum adjustments. When your partner can stay with you both day and night it helps him or her support and help you as well as begin to bond with the new baby and learn how to help meet the baby's needs.

Many hospitals have a room that respects cultural practices and allows smudging, for example. Hospitals will do their best to accommodate your culture and birth traditions.

Rooming in

In family-centred care, most babies "room in." This means mother and baby are not separated unless there is a medical problem. Babies stay in their mother's room. In most cases, it is healthy and best for mothers and their newborns to stay together from the moment of birth.

When an infant stays with the mother, the mother does most of the care, which reduces risk of infection from other babies and additional handling. Togetherness with the baby also helps a new mother to learn to recognize her baby's cues and respond to these in a timely way. Rooming in enables the mother to quickly meet the baby's breastfeeding needs.

Childbirth is a normal life experience, not an illness.

FAMILY-CENTRED CARE CHECKLIST

As you read the list put a check mark beside each statement that is true about your health care provider or birth location (hospital, birth centre, or home).

☐ *Will accept the birth plan I have prepared or has a standard birth plan I can change to suit my needs*

☐ *Will encourage me to have a labour support person in addition to my partner*

☐ *Welcomes skin-to-skin contact right after birth*

☐ *Encourages breastfeeding right after birth*

☐ *Will not separate my baby and me unless it is necessary for medical reasons*

☐ *Treats birth as a normal and natural process*

☐ *Will try to assign one nurse to me during my labour and birth (if possible)*

☐ *Accepts my religious beliefs and wants to do everything possible to meet my cultural needs*

☐ *Allows me to be part of decisions about procedures, labour positions, birth positions, and pain control*

(Continued)

Writing your birth plan

A birth plan enables you to consider your birth preferences and have them recorded in one place. This will allow for easy discussion with your health care provider and hospital staff. It may not always be possible to have everything go as you would have liked, but it helps to have thought through all the options in advance.

• What kind of childbirth would you like?
• How would you like your baby cared for after birth?

Many hospitals, birthing centres, and health care providers have a draft birth plan for you to use. You can also use the one provided by the Society of Obstetricians and Gynaecologists of Canada on their website: www.pregnancy.sogc.org/labour-and-childbirth/birth-plan/.

How to write a birth plan

Simple and short is best, usually less than one page long. Childbirth will include your health care team, yourself, your partner, the baby, and your family. Your birth plan works best if you write down what you want and what you would prefer if things do not happen as you planned. For example, you may write, "I would prefer not to have an intravenous line during labour. I will agree to have one if there is a clear medical reason."

When to write a birth plan

Most women write a birth plan after they talk over their childbirth plans with a health care provider and once they know what their hospital or birthing centre offers in terms of routines and care. It's also a good idea to discuss the plan with your partner and your family if they are going to be involved in some way. However, it is your body, and your family needs to understand that you are the only one who can make some of the more personal decisions (pain control, for example).

Common things included in a birth plan

These are some of the common things women include in their birth plans. You do not have to include all of them in your own birth plan. If something is not as important to you, you can leave it out. If you think of something else that is not on this list, feel free to include it.

No one can predict how your labour and birth will progress, so it is important to leave room for change. If someone from your health care team recommends a procedure, be sure to ask any questions that you may have and learn about the benefits, risks of doing or not doing the procedure, other options, and likely outcome.

The goal of birth is a healthy mother and a healthy baby.

Support during labour

Studies show that women who have a support person during their labour and birth often cope better with labour pain, use pain medication less often, need fewer medical interventions, have shorter labours, and see labour and birth as a positive experience. This person might be your partner, family member, friend, or a professional doula. They can work together with you and your health care team to help you during labour and birth and afterwards, too. If you give birth in a hospital, an obstetrical nurse will be present with you while you are in labour. In addition to providing for your medical needs, nurses are trained to provide labour support during labour and birth. Midwives also provide this support in hospitals, birthing centres, and during home births. Doulas are privately trained or experienced labour support persons who can provide you with extra continuous support during labour and birth. Doulas generally charge a fee for their service.

☐ *Has flexible visiting hours for close family members*

If you checked most of these boxes, your health care provider or birth location offers a family-friendly approach. Most health care workers will try very hard to meet your needs.

Enema and shaving

Today's health care providers do not usually recommend shaving a woman's pubic area or giving enemas to women in labour. An *enema* is a liquid put into the rectum to clear out the bowel. Some women find that having an enema gets rid of pressure in the lower bowel. This is most helpful if they were constipated before labour began.

Intravenous line (IV)

Sometimes an IV is the best way to give you certain medicines—such as antibiotics or drugs to start labour. Some women benefit from the extra fluids they can get through an IV if they are dehydrated and cannot tolerate oral fluids. If you want an epidural (see "Freezing (anaesthetics)" on page 162), you will need to have an IV.

Blood tests

If your pregnancy is thought to be low-risk, routine blood tests are not usually needed. Sometimes certain blood tests are needed (such as blood sugar tests if you are diabetic) to make sure all is going well.

Inducing labour

If your labour has not started by the end of your 41st week or if you have other medical problems, your health care provider may suggest that labour be *induced* (started using medical means). Labour should not be induced without good reason. (Read the section about overdue babies on page 139.)

Augmenting labour

If your labour is moving too slowly, your health care provider may suggest rupture of membranes or starting an IV with oxytocin. Oxytocin is a hormone that is almost the same as your natural labour hormone. It will cause the contractions to get stronger or become more regular.

Monitoring the baby

During normal labour, it is best to monitor the baby at regular intervals by listening to the baby's heart rate. This needs to happen in a way that does not limit your movements. If you have certain health concerns, it may be necessary to monitor the baby using continuous fetal monitoring, but this should be used only when needed (see "Monitoring your baby during labour" on page 151).

Movement during labour

Most hospitals, birth centres, and health care providers encourage mothers to move about freely during the early stages of labour because this helps speed up labour and helps you manage labour.

Eating and drinking during labour

In the early stages of labour, eating and drinking small amounts prevents you from becoming dehydrated and helps you keep up your strength. However, most women in active labour do not feel like eating. They may want to have small amounts of clear fluids. Some women with certain high-risk problems may not be allowed any food or drink.

Pain relief

There are many different ways to help you with the pain of labour and childbirth. These range from special breathing to an epidural block (if you choose). You can read more about ways to make labour easier in Chapter Six.

Pushing

At the end of active labour, the urge to push your baby out suddenly becomes strong. The body naturally wants to bear down (push) a few short times during each contraction. It is important to take breaths in and out between pushes. This way of pushing gives the baby the most oxygen. Sometimes, health care providers might ask you to push a different way. You may be encouraged to take a deep breath and hold it, then push one hard, long push with a deep breath at the end. This may speed up birth, but it may also lower the baby's oxygen levels over time.

Sometimes, the cervix is not quite ready for the baby to move through. You may be told not to push. If that happens, you will be told what you can do to avoid pushing (such as a knee-to-chest posture or special breathing).

Birth positions

The best position for birth is the one that is most comfortable for you. Some women prefer sitting upright or semi-sitting. Lying on your side is also a natural birth position that has many benefits. Squatting down can be helpful because it improves the angle of the pelvis, giving the baby more room to come out, and some women prefer to be kneeling on all fours.

Episiotomy

There is no evidence to support doing an *episiotomy* for all women (making a cut to widen the opening to the vagina). In fact, there are more benefits to *not* doing this:

- Less pain after the baby is born
- Better sexual function later
- Less relaxation of the pelvic muscles

In some cases, an episiotomy is necessary to relieve pressure or to assist with the birth of a baby in distress.

Religious or cultural beliefs

Feel free to list your needs in this area of your birth plan. You may have customs, beliefs, and certain things you want for yourself, the baby, and your family.

Rooming in

It is best for you and your new baby to stay and sleep in the same room. Babies who do so are handled mostly by their mothers. In most cases, it is healthy and best for mothers, partners, and their newborns to stay together from the moment of birth.

By rooming in, you and your baby have more time to bond with each other. Togetherness with the baby also helps a new mother and her partner to learn to recognize their baby's cues and respond to these in a timely way. Rooming in also enables the mother to quickly meet the baby's breastfeeding needs.

Examinations and procedures such as drawing blood should take place with mother and baby together. Breastfeeding and holding baby skin-to-skin are great ways to reduce baby's distress during painful procedures. Mothers and babies should be separated only for medical reasons and brought together as soon as possible.

Caesarean birth

If you know you will be having a caesarean birth, you may want to think about what kind of pain relief you want and if you want your partner to attend. If you need an emergency birth, what would your choices be? Include these in your birth plan.

Cutting the umbilical cord

"Cutting the cord" is a symbolic step, and many parents ask to make that part of their birth experience. Waiting at least 2 minutes after the baby is born before cutting the umbilical cord will help your baby get more blood and iron that will be needed in the

THE FOLLOWING WEBSITES PROVIDE MORE INFORMATION ON UMBILICAL CORD BLOOD BANKING:

• *Canadian Blood Services:*
www.blood.ca/cordblood

• *Héma-Québec:*
www.hema-quebec.qc.ca

Information is also available on private cord blood bank websites.

Your health care provider can advise you of the options in your community.

months to come. If your partner wishes to cut the cord, this can be arranged. If you have arranged for stem cell collection, check with the organization you are using for storage. Delayed cord clamping may affect the amount of blood available for storage.

Umbilical cord blood

Delayed cord clamping

After your baby is born, your doctor or nurse will wait before clamping the umbilical cord to allow your baby to get the iron that your baby will need during the first few months of life. Afterwards, the umbilical cord is cut and clamped; a length of umbilical cord is still linked to the placenta. This cord is filled with a small amount of blood, some of which is tested for the baby's blood type, haemoglobin level, and often for a test of the baby's level of pH (blood acidity) and oxygen. The rest of the blood is available for umbilical blood banking.

Umbilical cord blood banks

The blood in the umbilical cord contains special cells, called *stem cells,* which can be used to treat people with cancers such as leukaemia or lymphoma or other diseases of the blood cells. In other words, these cells could save someone's life.

If you choose to use or donate the umbilical cord blood, you should let your health care providers know now. There are forms to fill out and collection kits that need to be organized. Cord blood banks require that you go through a screening process before you reach 34 weeks. You need to include this in your birth plan. Umbilical cord blood must be taken after birth but before the placenta is delivered.

If you would like to collect and store your baby's cord blood you have some decisions to make now. There are private labs that will store the blood securely under your name for an annual cost, so that it would be available to you, for your child, or for subsequent children, if needed. And, similar to insurance, we all hope it will never be needed. Your health care provider can give you information on the labs that are available where you live.

You can also donate the cord blood to Canadian Blood Services, which collects voluntarily donated cord blood from mothers giving birth at designated hospitals across the country at no charge. Visit the Canadian Blood Services website to see where collection is possible and to download an information kit: www.blood.ca/cordblood. Canadian Blood Services tests and stores eligible blood stem cells from the umbilical cord and placenta and makes eligible cord blood units available for any patient in Canada or world-wide in need of an unrelated stem cell transplant.

Héma-Québec manages the only public cord bank in Québec. There are several partner hospitals where women planning to give birth can register. This is linked to the Canadian registry as well: www.hema-quebec.qc.ca/cellules-souches/don-sang-cordon-ombilical/index.en.html.

Skin-to-skin contact

Uninterrupted skin-to-skin contact with your baby right after birth for at least the first hour or until the baby has breastfed or for as long as the mother wishes is important. Being skin-to-skin with your baby helps your baby adjust to life outside the womb, helps bonding, and is a good time to begin breastfeeding. If there is a medical reason for the mother not to do so, a partner or support person can hold the baby skin-to-skin until the mother is stable and can have the baby skin-to-skin with her. If baby is not able to be skin-to-skin at birth, start spending time skin-to-skin as soon as you can. Skin-to-skin is important for all babies regardless of how the baby will be fed.

Starting to breastfeed

Studies show that being skin-to-skin with your baby makes it easier for your baby to begin breastfeeding. Babies have natural instincts that enable them to know how to breastfeed when they are skin-to-skin. They will often seek the breast and show signs of wanting to feed such as rooting, licking their lips, and making sucking motions. Some babies latch onto the breast and feed. Some medications and procedures used during labour and birth can affect the initiation of breastfeeding. Start being skin-to-skin with baby as soon as you can, and this will help your baby learn to breastfeed.

Breastfeeding after a caesarean birth

Many mothers and babies are able to enjoy being skin-to-skin immediately or soon after a caesarean birth as long as a general anaesthetic was not needed. If the mother is not available (too groggy, etc.), baby can be placed skin-to-skin with a person of the mother's choosing such as her partner or support person. Breastfeeding after a caesarean birth is very common. If for some reason the baby cannot go to the breast soon after the birth, hand expression can help initiate breastfeeding.

Feeding your baby

Your baby isn't here yet—but this is the right time to begin planning.

Breastfeeding is an important choice for both the baby and mother. The Society of Obstetricians and Gynaecologists of Canada (SOGC), the Canadian Paediatric Society (CPS), Dietitians of Canada (DC), Health Canada, the World Health Organization (WHO), and the United Nations Children's Fund (UNICEF) recommend exclusive breastfeeding for the first 6 months of life and continued breastfeeding up to age 2 and beyond. After 6 months of only breastfeeding, and based on your baby's signs of readiness, you can begin to introduce solid foods to your baby. Start with iron-rich foods such as meats, poultry, fish, eggs, tofu, legumes (beans, lentils, and chickpeas), and fortified infant cereals. For more information on feeding solids to your baby, visit www.healthycanadians.gc.ca/healthy-living-vie-saine/infant-care-soins-bebe/nutrition-alimentation-eng.php.

When to feed: knowing the signs

Studies show it is best to breastfeed when your baby shows early signs of hunger such as stirring, mouth opening, rooting, and hands, fists, or fingers to the mouth. Waiting until your baby shows later signs of hunger, such as crying, can make feeding more difficult. These signs are called *cues*. Staying together with your baby will help you to know and understand your baby's early hunger signs and allow you to respond quickly. Babies should feed at least eight times during a 24-hour period. Babies need to be fed at night as well as during the day. If your baby is feeding fewer than eight times in 24 hours, you may need to wake him to feed. Talk to your health care provider.

Just breast milk

Studies show that breastfed babies aged 0–6 months do not need feedings of anything other than breast milk. Water feedings are not necessary.

Asking for help

Always ask for help. Many places and many people can help with breastfeeding (hospital, birth centre, public health nurses, midwives, breastfeeding clinics, or professional breastfeeding experts, called *lactation consultants,* and even other mothers).

Most babies are ready to breastfeed within the first hour after they are born. Until your milk volume increases (usually 2 to 4 days after the birth), your breasts will produce the first milk called colostrum. This colostrum has antibodies, omega-3 fatty acids, and the perfect balance of nutrients, minerals, vitamins, and trace elements for your baby.

The colostrum feedings are perfect for your baby and all she needs at this time.

Most babies lose weight after birth and use the fat and water stored in their bodies. This weight loss should not be more than 7% of their birth weight in the first 2 to 4 days after birth, and they should regain the lost weight in about 2 weeks. If you are concerned about your baby's weight loss, you should speak with your health care provider.

It is best to breastfeed your newborn whenever he shows signs of being hungry (sucking on his fist, smacking his lips, trying to suck on anything near him). Babies should not be given water.

Breastfeeding—the natural and healthy way to feed your baby

The importance of breastfeeding for baby and mother is well-recognized. Breast milk is made just for your baby. Breastfeeding helps protect babies against infectious diseases, sudden infant death syndrome, and may also have a protective effect against obesity. For mothers, breastfeeding can delay menstruation and it may reduce the risk of chronic diseases, such as ovarian and breast cancers.

Today, nearly 90% of Canadian mothers start to breastfeed; however, only one-quarter of them breastfeed exclusively for the recommended 6 months. Exclusive breastfeeding means baby gets breast milk and no other liquids or solids. Breast milk, including the first milk that your breasts produce (colostrum), contains antibodies that complete your baby's immune system and help fight disease. A strong immune system lowers the chance of your baby getting infections.

Breast milk is easily digested and breastfed babies rarely have problems with stomach upset or constipation. Babies are hardly ever allergic to breast milk. Breast milk also contains active proteins that support the development of your baby's gut, nerves, and disease-fighting cells.

Talk to other women and to organizations such as the La Leche League Canada Breastfeeding Referral Service (1-800-665-4324) or your local public health nurse to learn more. Most hospitals have staff who have had special training to help you with breastfeeding. In some places, breastfeeding clinics and private breastfeeding experts are also available.

Most mothers are able to breastfeed. Sometimes mothers who want to breastfeed need to give their babies infant formula for a medical reason and some mothers decide to give formula for personal reasons. It is always important to get the information that you need to make an informed decision. Talk to your health care provider, who will help with the current best information and support you with the decision you make. See "Feeding your baby" on page 219 for more information on feeding your baby.

Breastfeeding myths—true and false

1. Breastfeeding is easy, natural, and based on human instinct.

   True. Once you and your baby have started and then developed your own routine, breastfeeding is easy and the most natural way to feed a baby. Similar to many new things, it can take time to get it right. Be patient with yourself. Ask for help. Stay with your decision—it's worth it.

2. I shouldn't start breastfeeding because I'm not sure I can continue for more than 2 or 3 months.

   False. It is important for your baby to be breastfed for any amount of time, even if it's just for a few days. This way, your baby will get the advantages of your milk and you will be able to keep your options open. Even if you do not know how long you will be able to breastfeed, it is important to start.

3. Mothers who breastfeed are "tied" to their babies.

   True. But then, all new mothers are "tied" to their babies. Breastfeeding or not, your newborn will need frequent feedings and care. Yes, breastfeeding mothers do need to stay close to their babies, which is natural. You will feel good knowing that you are there to breastfeed and comfort your baby. Unlike formula, no additional time or special preparations are required for breastfeeding. In the early months, take the baby with you. Mothers have the right to breastfeed their babies in a public place. You will likely find breastfeeding offers you both convenience and flexibility. Some new mothers feel lonely and miss the regular contact with other adults. Many communities have mother-to-mother support groups and breastfeeding support groups such as La Leche League. Talk to your health care provider or visit a health centre to ask about the support available in your community.

4. Most women can produce enough milk to feed their baby.

True. Breastfeeding your baby promotes your body's milk supply so you can meet your baby's exact demands. Sometimes a mother thinks she is not producing enough milk. In most cases, problems can be resolved with help from a person trained in breastfeeding. If you have concerns, talk to your health care provider or find a program in your community that supports breastfeeding mothers.

5. Babies must suck in a different way from a bottle than from a breast.

True. Babies who are bottle-fed need to learn a different type of sucking than breastfed babies. Some babies become confused by the difference between your nipple and the nipple of a bottle. Other babies develop a preference for the firmness or flow of an artificial nipple. This can cause nipple confusion and nipple preference and can lead to a baby refusing to breastfeed. Pacifier use can also interfere with breastfeeding.

6. If I breastfeed, I should not bottle feed at all.

Many breastfed babies never receive a bottle. Sucking on a bottle nipple or pacifier is different than sucking at breast. Babies sometimes become confused or learn to prefer the firmness of a bottle nipple. Also, the way your body produces milk will match your baby's demand when you respond to your baby's hunger cues by breastfeeding. If you need to be separated from your baby there are many methods that you can try. Your expressed or pumped milk can be fed to your baby. A dropper or syringe can be used for small amounts and otherwise a cup or finger feeding are other options that can be used. Talk to someone experienced with helping breastfeeding mothers and learn about the different methods before you make a decision. Studies show that giving your baby a bottle with an artificial nipple raises the chance that the baby will be weaned (stop breastfeeding) early.

7. Children should be weaned at 6 months of age.

    False. Breast milk is the best milk for babies and toddlers. The World Health Organization (WHO) and Health Canada recommend only breastfeeding for the first 6 months of life and continued breastfeeding for up to 2 years and beyond. Breastfeed for as long as you and your child wish.

8. Some mothers should not breastfeed.

    Rare, but this can be true. There are some medical conditions when breastfeeding is not recommended. Also, a health care provider may advise a woman not to breastfeed if a medication she is using could harm the baby. Most medications are compatible with breastfeeding. Talk to your health care provider about breastfeeding and any medicines that you take.

9. Women with breast implants cannot breastfeed.

    False. Many women with implants can breastfeed.

10. Blue or watery breast milk has no nutritional value.

    False. The odor and colour of human milk can vary. All breast milk has nutritional value for your baby.

11. The small amount of colostrum is enough for your baby in the first few days.

    True. Colostrum provides both water and sugar, as well as protein, minerals, and important antibodies that your baby cannot get from anything but breast milk.

12. Breastfed babies should be given a soother (pacifier) to help them learn to suck.

   False. A soother may teach your baby poor sucking technique. It may hide the baby's hunger signs from you and it can spread infection. There are many ways to soothe a fussy baby including skin-to-skin contact.

13. It is best to breastfeed a baby whenever she seems hungry.

   True. Breastfeeding your baby on cue makes for a more satisfied baby and success with breastfeeding. Most babies feed at least eight times during a 24-hour period.

14. Breastfed babies need to have water.

   False. Breast milk contains enough water to meet your baby's needs. Water has no nutritional value, and feeding your baby water can make your baby less hungry at feeding time.

15. If I breastfeed, I should eat well.

   Everyone should eat well and follow the *Eating Well with Canada's Food Guide* for their own health and well-being. Breastfeeding women need more calories. These can be met by including an extra two to three Food Guide servings each day. Eating well helps you recover from the baby's birth and helps your body heal. If you are not eating a healthy diet, breastfeeding is still the best way to feed your baby.

16. I have to wean my baby before I go back to work.

   False. Mothers who return to work have several choices. Some mothers breastfeed when they are at home and express their milk while at work for their baby to have the next day. Sometimes it is possible for their baby to be brought to the workplace to breastfeed. Please see www.chrc-ccdp.gc.ca/eng/content/policy-and-best-practices-page-2 to learn more about your rights as a breastfeeding mother to be accommodated at work.

My pregnancy journal
26 to 32 weeks

During your prenatal visit, your health care provider will weigh and measure you and your baby. Your health care provider will discuss the signs of preterm labour with you and how you are reducing the risks. Are you eating well and getting regular exercise? Are you protecting your baby from cigarette smoke and alcohol? Is your work stressful or does it make you very tired? Do you get enough rest?

If you have had any tests or a screening ultrasound since your last visit, your health care provider will review the results with you.

Together, you will also review your plans for childbirth and what you can expect. Talking about these things, combined with the reading you are doing, will help you get a clear picture of the choices you have for birthing your baby. You will start to think about how you want to proceed, based on what you think is best for you, your baby, and your partner.

KEEPING TRACK OF MY PROGRESS

Date:

Week of pregnancy:

Blood pressure:

Weight:

THINGS TO DISCUSS WITH MY HEALTH CARE PROVIDER

Questions about breastfeeding:

Questions about my birth plan:

Weight gain/nutrition:

Other concerns:

Date:

Week of pregnancy:

Blood pressure:

Weight:

Questions about breastfeeding:

Questions about my birth plan:

Weight gain/nutrition:

Other concerns:

My pregnancy journal
32 to 36 weeks

You will have prenatal visits every 2 to 3 weeks. Both you and your baby will be weighed and measured and your health care provider will continue to look for any signs of preterm labour. Your baby's health and growth will be the focus of these visits.

You and your health care provider will review your birth plan at this visit (see "Writing your birth plan" on page 116) and talk about any concerns you may have about childbirth.

Eating well is still very important, because your baby is growing quickly.

My to-do list

_____

_____

_____

_____

_____

_____

_____

_____

_____

_____

_____

_____

_____

_____

_____

_____

_____

_____

_____

_____

_____

_____

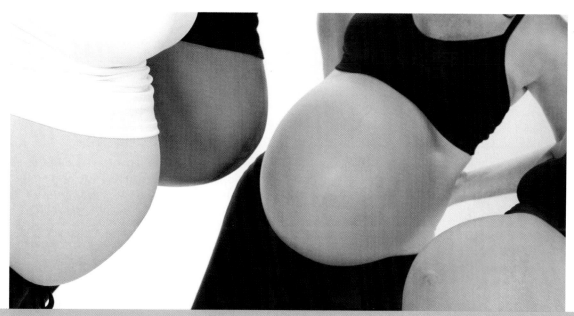

CHAPTER FIVE

Getting ready for baby's birth

**IMPORTANT THINGS TO THINK
ABOUT BEFORE LABOUR BEGINS**

- *How will you contact your labour support partner when you are ready?*

- *Do you have an alternate person you can contact?*

  If you are planning to give birth at a hospital or birthing centre:

- *Who will drive you there? You should not drive during labour. You will need to focus on yourself. If you plan to take a taxi, make sure you have taxi money. Contact social services if you need funds to help you get to the hospital.*

- *How far are you from the hospital? It is best to drive the distance before labour and record how long it takes to make the journey.*

- *What if road conditions are bad, the weather is bad, or if you must travel during rush hour traffic? Plan different routes to avoid any problems you can think of.*

(Continued)

Welcome to your final checklist before childbirth! Labour usually begins between the 37th and 42nd week of pregnancy. It is best to be prepared for labour. We'll talk about common discomforts near the end of your pregnancy, overdue babies, and the difference between pre-labour and true labour. The end of your pregnancy is near and you are very close to holding the newest member of your family.

Your changing body

Your pelvic bones have loosened and may ache, especially at the back. You may notice your breasts leaking some colostrum, leaving a thin crust on your nipples (not all women leak colostrum before the baby is born). Your breasts may feel full and heavy. Your belly may become so stretched that your navel pushes out. Near the end of your pregnancy, you may notice that the colour of your skin (pigmentation) looks browner and becomes darker.

Your uterus will begin to "practise" contractions (also called *Braxton Hicks contractions*) that may or may not be painless and are irregular. Because the uterus is putting a lot of pressure on the blood vessels in your pelvis, you may notice more swelling in your feet and ankles, which is common.

Near the end of pregnancy, most babies will settle into the head down, or "engaged," position. The event is sometimes known as "when the baby drops" or "lightening." However, in most cases engagement occurs as a gradual process. For some women, this does not happen until just before labour starts, which is also normal.

When your baby settles into your pelvis, the head will rest inside the pelvic bones. You will feel different and it will appear that you are carrying the baby much lower than you were before. After the baby settles into the pelvis, breathing will be easier. Sometimes, the lower heavy weight can add to a feeling of muscle strain and backache.

Your baby at full term

Your full-term baby is fully grown and measures 46–51 cm (18–20 in) in length and weighs between 3 and 4 kg (6.5 to 9 lbs).

Your baby's eyes are open when awake and closed when sleeping. Her lungs are now producing a substance called *surfactant* that will help her take the first breath. The placenta now measures about 20 cm (8–10 in) across and is about 2.5 cm (1 in) thick.

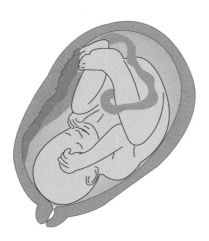

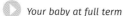 *Your baby at full term*

IMPORTANT THINGS TO THINK ABOUT BEFORE LABOUR BEGINS (CONTINUED)

- *Where are you supposed to park the car? Do you need to pre-register at the hospital or can you just arrive?*

- *Who will take care of your children at home?*

- *Do you need someone to feed your pets while you are away?*

- *Create your "Labour action list" and "Contact list" (see pages 251 and 252).*

- *Collect supplies recommended by your midwife if you are planning a home birth.*

- *If you are planning to keep your placenta, make sure that you have necessary supplies and you have informed your health care provider. You will likely need to sign a form when you bring it home.*

If you are giving birth at a hospital or birthing centre, pack a bag a few weeks before your due date, in case your baby arrives early. Your hospital or birthing centre may have a list of suggested items to pack. Once labour begins, you may not have time to pack everything you want to take with you.

PACKING CHECKLIST FOR YOU

☐ *This book, pen, and paper*
☐ *Copy of your birth plan if you have one*
☐ *Housecoat, nightgown, and slippers*
☐ *Loose-fitting clothing to go home in*
☐ *Extra pair of socks*
☐ *Bra (breastfeeding or good support bra)*
☐ *Underwear*
☐ *Sanitary napkins*
☐ *Toothbrush and toothpaste*
☐ *Hairbrush, comb*
☐ *Camera and batteries*
☐ *Charging cables and plugs or spare battery packs for any electronics that you may be bringing with you*
☐ *Coins for vending machines*
☐ *Labour-support items, such as massage oil for back rubs and tennis balls*

(Continued)

Common discomforts in late pregnancy

As they get closer to 40 weeks of pregnancy, many women begin to feel ready to have the baby—they are feeling the pressure from the baby in their back and their pelvis, they may have started to waddle, and their body is telling them it is time!

Difficulties sleeping

Sleeping difficulties are common throughout pregnancy but most common in the final trimester. Your enlarged belly makes it hard to find a comfortable position, and the added trips to the bathroom at night do not help either. Try using two or three large pillows to support your legs, belly, and back. A back massage may help you drift off to sleep. It may help to take a warm bath before going to bed. Try keeping the bedroom temperature cool. Do not take sleeping pills unless your health care provider approves them. Avoid caffeine and eat your evening meal several hours before bedtime. You may find meditation and mindfulness exercises helpful.

Discharge from your vagina

Discharge from your vagina usually increases during pregnancy. During your last trimester, it can become even more plentiful.

Discharge should be:

- Clear
- Sticky
- Odourless

If your discharge is thick and white or bloody, your mucous plug may have released and your cervix may have begun opening. If it is watery, you could be leaking amniotic fluid, meaning that your water bag has broken. If your discharge has a foul odour, you may have an infection. You should not feel any pain, itching, or soreness in your vaginal area. Contact your health care provider if you have any of these signs.

Pre-labour contractions

Pre-labour contractions (Braxton Hicks contractions) are usually light and painless and do not occur in any regular pattern. They're normal and are thought to be the muscles of your uterus preparing for labour. Many women do not even notice when they happen. They are different from the contractions that come with labour—which begin slowly and then become more frequent, stronger, and regular. Refer to the below information about "true labour" and "pre-labour." If you think you may be in labour, contact a health care provider.

Overdue babies

About 10% of women will not give birth to their babies by the end of their 41st week, or within 1 week after their due date. When a pregnancy goes beyond that, it is called **post-term** and the baby is said to be **overdue.** To be sure your pregnancy is truly post-term, your baby's due date must be accurate. Your due date will have been calculated early in your pregnancy using the date of your last menstrual period and the results of the earliest ultrasound of your pregnancy. Trying to calculate due dates late in pregnancy using uncertain menstrual dates or late ultrasounds is not reliable.

PACKING YOUR SUITCASE
(CONTINUED)

☐ *You may prefer your own pillow to hospital pillows. If you do bring your own, use a colorful pillow case to prevent mix-ups.*

PACKING CHECKLIST FOR
YOUR BABY

☐ *Clothing to go home in*
☐ *Diapers and wipes*
☐ *Receiving blanket*
☐ *Warmer blanket*
☐ *Hat*
☐ *Car seat*
☐ *Your hospital may recommend additional items.*

TRUE LABOUR VERSUS PRE-LABOUR

True labour means labour pains that become regular and lead to childbirth. There may be a few "false starts" that feel just like true labour, but then stop. Each one of those contractions is not wasted but is helping to ready your body for birthing. If you do not know whether you are in true labour, it's helpful to time the contractions and note how strong and regular they are. Write down how many minutes apart they are, from the start of one contraction until the start of the next, and note how long each one lasts. If possible, keep a record for 1 hour.

1. HOW STRONG ARE THE CONTRACTIONS?

TRUE LABOUR

• *The contractions will gradually get stronger over time.*

• *You will be able to feel your uterus becoming firmer.*

PRE-LABOUR

• *The contractions do not gradually get stronger over time.*

• *They may weaken at times and even go away for a while.*

2. IS YOUR CERVIX CHANGING?

TRUE LABOUR

• *Your cervix begins to change as it softens, shortens, and opens.*

• *If the cervix opens to 3 or 4 cm (about 1.2 to 1.6 in) with regular contractions, this is a sign of active labour.*

PRE-LABOUR

• *There is no change in your cervix.*

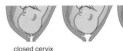

closed cervix   open cervix

• *It does not soften, shorten, thin out, or open up.*

TRUE LABOUR VERSUS PRE-LABOUR (CONTINUED)

3. HOW REGULAR ARE THE CONTRACTIONS?

True labour
- *The contractions usually become quite regular. You can predict them.*

- *In true labour, contractions last 30 to 70 seconds and are about 5 minutes apart (or less).*

PRE-LABOUR
- *The contractions are not regular and never really settle down into a pattern.*

An aging placenta

A small number of overdue babies will develop health issues. We do not know why some overdue babies have these problems, but it may be because of an aging placenta. As it gets older, the placenta begins to lose its ability to do its job. When this happens, it may mean that fewer nutrients and less blood and oxygen reach your baby. In some cases, this can cause stress for your baby and slow his growth.

Making sure your overdue baby is safe

If your baby is overdue, your health care provider will be keeping a very close watch on your baby. You can keep close track of how the baby is doing by counting the baby's movements (see page 111). It may also be recommended that you have a test that measures the fetal heart rate (non-stress testing) as well as an ultrasound that measures the baby's well-being and the amount of amniotic fluid. Your health care provider will discuss this with you and arrange any further testing that may be suggested. You and your health care provider will discuss whether or not to induce labour (see Chapter Six for many more details).

KEEPING TRACK OF MY PROGRESS

Date:

Week of pregnancy:

Blood pressure:

Weight:

THINGS TO DISCUSS WITH MY HEALTH CARE PROVIDER

My pregnancy journal
36 to 42 weeks

You will have prenatal visits every week during the last 4 to 6 weeks of your pregnancy. At each visit, your health care provider will examine both you and your baby closely. The goal is to make sure that you are both making good progress and that your body is getting ready for the big event: childbirth.

My to-do list

Your time is here

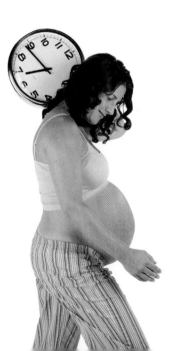

With twins or multiples, your labour experience may be slightly different from what is described in this chapter. You likely already have discussed what to expect with your health care provider or a specialist. This chapter will help you with the basics of labour and birth.

Go to the hospital or birth centre when one or more of the following occurs:

- *Your water breaks in a gush or is leaking steadily.*

- *Your contractions are regular and 5 minutes apart (and the hospital or birth centre is less than 30 minutes away).*

- *Your contractions are regular and 10 minutes apart (and the hospital or birth centre is more than 30 minutes away).*

You have arrived at the moment everyone has been waiting for—the start of labour. In this chapter, we'll discuss the signs of labour, followed by the four stages of labour. We'll talk about your "water breaking," breathing, positions, pain relief, and assisted birth techniques. We also have included a section on bonding with your baby.

Because sometimes things do not go as planned, we talk about interventions that you may need to keep you and your baby safe during labour and birth.

So, after months of waiting (and maybe when you least expect it), you'll begin to feel the start of labour. Similar to most women, you may feel surprised, excited, and even a little afraid. But yours is the major role in the final act of this 9-month miracle—the growth of a fertilized egg that was smaller than the dot over the *i* in the word *life* into a living, breathing human being. You are about to experience the joy of bringing a new life into your family.

When labour begins

No one can predict when your labour will begin. There is no single thing that prompts labour, although we think hormones play an important role. So, this section will prepare you for the signs of labour and help you to be ready to respond.

If you are not sure what to do or how to measure your contractions, call the labour and birthing unit at your hospital, the birthing centre, or your health care provider. If you are under midwifery care, you will be given instructions for whom and when to call when you are experiencing signs of labour.

Signs of labour

Some women know they are in labour right away. Others may not be so sure. Sometimes, it is even hard for your health care provider to know. If you are in doubt, you should contact your health care provider or go to the hospital or birth centre to be assessed.

Mucous plug: During your pregnancy, a mucous plug forms at the opening of your cervix. When your cervix begins to open (or dilate), this plug is released. This plug is a large clump of thick mucous or increased mucous discharge that may have streaks of blood in it. This may happen many days before labour starts, so you may need to wait for other signs that labour has begun.

Bloody show: Bloody show is the result of blood being released from capillaries when the cervix starts to thin and open. It may look pink or light red. It is an early sign of labour. If you have bright red bleeding, you should go to your place of birth to be assessed.

Ruptured membrane: You may have heard the expression that your "water will break." The medical term is *ruptured membrane*. Both refer to the same thing: when the sac of amniotic fluid around your baby begins leaking or breaks open fully. This can happen many hours before labour begins or at any time during labour. Go to the hospital when this happens whether or not labour contractions have started.

Contractions: Labour often begins with contractions of the uterus, when your uterus gets tight and then relaxes. These contractions happen so that your cervix will open and help move the baby down the birth canal. (See pages 140 and 141 to learn the difference between true labour and pre-labour.)

True labour contractions are painful and regular, and they usually last somewhere between 30 and 70 seconds.

I'M HAVING CONTRACTIONS—IS THIS LABOUR?

A number of factors will help you determine if you're in labour—when in doubt, you should contact or see a health care provider.

Once you experience contractions, the key factors to consider (and write down) are as follows:

- *Frequency of contractions—time and record your contractions, from the start of one contraction to the start of the next contraction, as well as how long they last, for example, occur 10 minutes apart and last 30 seconds.*

- *Strength of contractions—how strong are they? Can you feel your uterus actually becoming "hard," and are the contractions causing discomfort or pain (usually in the lower abdomen or back)?*

- *Duration—for how long have you been having the contractions, that is, have you been having them for a couple of hours, all afternoon, or . . . ?*

The importance of labour support

You can count on having the support of your health care team in labour, but you may feel more confident if you have someone to provide extra support with you. Choose someone you trust, who makes you feel comfortable, and who will be able to encourage you and make your wishes known while you are in labour.

A support person is usually someone other than a health care provider. A support person can be any of the following people: your partner, a relative, a friend, or a doula.

A doula is a person who has taken some extra training to support a women and her partner before, during, and after birth. They can be an important support person, and be available in addition to your other support people. The training can be variable (a weekend course to 2 to 3 months of training). Hiring a doula is a personal choice and is not publicly funded.

Helping your support person prepare

Support people need to prepare, especially if this is their first birth. They may wonder how they will help during labour. Some may worry about feeling nervous or queasy and not being able to offer enough support.

Here are a few suggestions for your labour support person:
- It is okay to feel a bit nervous, especially if this is the first time you are supporting someone in labour.
- Your presence alone can make a big difference for the labouring woman. You don't always have to be "doing something" to be supportive.
- Before labour begins, you can help with household chores and encourage the pregnant woman to rest.
- Become familiar with her birth plan so that you can be her advocate during labour and birth.

- During labour, you can help by being calm. You can offer words of encouragement and help the labouring woman to relax between contractions.
- Follow her lead when helping her with her breathing. Her body often tells her which rhythm is best.
- If she feels like she is losing control, you can help by talking her quietly through the contraction and maintaining eye contact. Between contractions you can talk about ways that may help her cope better, such as using massage or changing positions, or just let her rest.
- Be flexible. Things don't always go as planned, and the labouring woman may also change her mind about how she wants to manage her pain. If she changes her mind, you must remind yourself that she is the one in labour and it is always her choice to make.
- Remember to take care of yourself during labour. Take time to eat, drink, and rest.

Your labour and birthing team

You may decide to give birth in a hospital, birthing centre, or at home. In most cases, hospital births begin with meeting your obstetrical nurse when you arrive. Most labour and birthing professionals are registered nurses, but some may have training as midwives. When possible, the same nurse will stay with you during your labour and birth. Licensed midwives also care for women during pregnancy, labour, and birth, both in hospital and in other settings.

Studies show that you will benefit from having a nurse or midwife who is focused on your care. These partners want to help you master techniques to make your labour easier. They are also very experienced and know when the birth process is going well and when it is not.

The stages of labour

There are four stages of labour:
- Stage 1 begins with the first contractions, when they become regular. It ends when your cervix is fully open (dilated) at 10 centimetres.
- Stage 2 begins when your cervix is fully open (dilated) and ends when your baby is born.
- Stage 3 begins after the baby is born and ends when the placenta is delivered.
- Stage 4 is the immediate time after the birth during which the mother starts her recovery from the birth.

The average time for labour is 12 to 14 hours for a first childbirth. Labour is often shorter for women who have already had a baby. Keep in mind that these are just averages and that every labour is different. No one can predict what your labour will be like or how long it will last.

Early in pregnancy, your cervix is a thick-walled canal about 2.5 cm (1 in) long. It is closed. During the last few weeks of your pregnancy, hormones will make your cervix soften. This is called the **ripening** of the cervix. Once labour begins, contractions make the ripened cervix **efface** (thin out) and **dilate** (open up). At the end of the first stage of labour, your cervix will be open 10 centimetres (4 inches) and the sides will be very thin. At this point, your uterus, cervix, and vagina will shape themselves into one continuous birth canal for the baby to pass through.

The first stage of labour

The first stage of labour usually lasts the longest. It is divided into three parts: early, active, and transition.

MONITORING YOUR BABY DURING LABOUR

In a low-risk pregnancy, the best way to check on a baby's well-being during labour is to listen to its heart through the mother's belly. A nurse or midwife will check the fetal heart rate often and regularly by using a stethoscope or a hand-held Doppler (an ultrasound machine that picks up the sounds of your baby's heart).

During labour, the fetal heart rate will be checked at these intervals:

- *For a full minute after a contraction about two to four times each hour during the first stage of labour*

- *Every 5 minutes when you begin the second stage of labour and start pushing*

If your pregnancy or labour is considered high-risk, or if a problem arises during labour, your health care team may need to use some form of electronic fetal monitoring to know how your baby is doing, especially during the contractions. This type of monitor is often used in the following situations:

- *Your baby's heart rate is too slow or too fast*

- *The baby has had a bowel movement known as* meconium *(the first stool that a baby passes) while still in the uterus*

Fetal monitoring using electronic fetal monitoring is very common, but it should only be used if there are concerns about the baby's heart rate or if the mother has known medical risks. It limits a mother's ability to walk around or move freely during labour, unless wireless monitoring is available. The monitor can measure and record a baby's heartbeat and the length and strength of the mother's contractions.

Sometimes it is necessary to take a sample of blood from the baby's scalp (fetal scalp sampling) to check blood oxygen and pH levels.

External monitor	Internal monitor
The mother wears a belt around her belly.	A small electrode attached to a monitor is inserted through the mother's vagina.
The belt has wires that are attached to the monitor.	A scalp clip is attached to a part of the baby that can be reached through the open cervix (usually the top of the head).

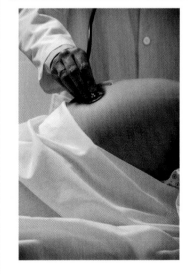

Slow progress in labour is common. If this is your first childbirth, the time from the start of active labour to birth averages about 12 to 14 hours.

If dilation is slow you may be given oxytocin, a synthetic hormone, to make your contractions stronger and more frequent. Oxytocin can help with a slow labour in two ways:

- *It prevents labour from going on for too long (exhausting the mother and putting stress on the baby).*

- *It reduces the need for a caesarean birth.*

Early (or latent) stage: 0–3 cm

In this early stage, it may be hard to know for sure if you are in labour. Tracking the strength and regularity of your contractions and paying close attention to any changes to your cervix will determine if you are in labour. If you go to the hospital during this stage, you will be assessed and then may be observed for a few hours or told to go home until labour is well established.

During this latent or early part of labour, eat a light meal, drink fluids, and try a warm bath or a shower. Sometimes, if you have been having irregular contractions and you are tired, you may be offered some pain medicine to help you rest and regain your strength for when labour gets stronger.

Active stage: 3–8 cm

You will notice that your contractions have become much stronger. They last about 45 seconds and occur about every 3 to 5 minutes. As the contractions progress, your cervix will continue to thin and open. At the end of this stage, your cervix will have opened to 8 centimetres. You may experience many emotions . . . all are normal. Try to relax between contractions. Try breathing techniques to focus and manage the contractions. You may begin to feel quite tired, so rest and recover as much as you can between contractions. You may have some back pain because of where your baby's head is sitting in your pelvis.

Transition stage: 8–10 cm

You are almost at the end of Stage 1 now. Your contractions may be every 2 to 3 minutes and will usually last about 60 to 90 seconds. This helps your cervix to dilate fully to 10 centimetres. In many women, labour actually slows down during the transition stage, and it may take longer to dilate the final 2 centimetres. While your cervix dilates these last couple of centimetres, your baby's head should be moving down slowly into your pelvis.

Medication-free ways to make labour easier

Labour tends to be easier if you are relaxed and feel confident. Many of the techniques that you and your support team will use to make labour easier, will also help you relax and remain in control of your body and mind.

You and your support person will have learned and practised many different techniques in the weeks and months before labour began. Remember, a technique that works for other women may not work for you. That's why it's good to know as many techniques as possible.

Special breathing

The way you breathe during labour may help make your job easier and give you a sense of control over your body and mind. Sometimes you will just follow your body's lead and breathe in the way that feels right for you. You may also find some of the three following techniques helpful.

Slow breathing

Slow, deep breathing works best in the early stage of labour because it shifts your focus away from the contractions. Begin by taking a deep breath through your nose or mouth. Then purse your lips as if you are blowing up a balloon and very slowly blow the air out. For many women, the rate and rhythm of this kind of breathing comes naturally, but a handy rule is to breathe in for three or four counts and then out for three or four counts. Many women in labour find that this type of slow breathing helps them all the way through their entire labour.

Light/quick breathing

This type of breathing works best during the active part of labour, when the contractions are coming more often and are getting quite strong. When a contraction begins, start by breathing slowly in and out. As the contraction gets stronger, shorten your breaths. At the peak of the contraction (the strongest point), breathe lightly in and quickly out, making a puffing sound almost like a dog panting. When the contraction starts to ease off, slow your breathing down again and then take a deep, cleansing breath.

Transition breathing (pant-pant-blow)

During the transition stage of labour—when the labour is most intense and you find it hard to breathe slowly—this kind of breathing can help you resist the urge to push against a cervix that is not fully dilated. It is often called "pant-pant-blow breathing" and is done by taking a deep breath in, then exhaling two short pants, followed by a longer blow to empty your lungs.

Coping with early labour	
You can	*Your support person can*
• Take a warm bath or a shower.	• Put your bags into the car if you are giving birth at a hospital or birthing centre.
• Walk with your support person or watch a movie.	• Help you relax by offering you a back or foot massage.
• Use relaxation techniques.	• Let people know labour has started, if necessary.
• Breathe slowly and deeply through contractions.	• Encourage you to walk, rest, eat, and drink.
• Keep your energy levels up by eating and drinking lightly.	• Time your contractions from the start of one to the start of the next.
	• Be calm and reassuring.
	• Prepare a light meal for you and offer you plenty of fluids.

Coping with active labour	
You can	*Your support person can*
• *Relax; go with the flow of contractions.*	• *Massage tense muscles.*
• *Use light/quick breathing or a slow relaxed breathing.*	• *Stay with you.*
• *Change positions often. Moving will speed up labour.*	• *Help with your breathing, letting your rhythm dictate the best breathing pattern for you.*
• *Expect your contractions to get much stronger after your water breaks.*	• *Encourage and help you to change positions often. Use pillows for support. Walk with you. Help you to sit up if that's what you want to do.*
• *Ask for pain relief if you need it.*	• *Apply firm counter-pressure to your back during contractions. Give back massages between contractions.*
• *Use visualization to help you to focus.*	• *Be your voice with your doctor, midwife, or nurse.*
• *Take a warm bath or a shower.*	• *Let you focus on your labour.*
• *Use a birthing ball to put counter-pressure on your perineum and to help open up your pelvis.*	• *Encourage you and tell you how far you have come. Help you get through contractions one at a time and prepare for the next one.*
• *Ask for help; make your needs known.*	• *Support your choices. Never criticize. Make the room as peaceful as possible. Be calm and reassuring.*

Coping with the transition to second-stage labour	
You can	*Your labour coach can*
• Move around as much as you need to get comfortable.	• Support your choice of position.
• Try the pant-pant-blow breathing to help resist the urge to push if your cervix is not dilated to 10 centimetres.	• Help with breathing. Maintain eye contact so that you feel linked to someone and more in control.
• Get through your contractions one at a time.	• Remind you that labour is almost over and the baby is nearly out. Be calm and offer positive support.
• Visualize your body opening up like a flower to let your baby move out.	• Rub tense muscles if you want, especially around the lower back where the baby's head may be applying pressure.
• Rest in between contractions.	• Help you with visualization and relaxation.
• Use a cool cloth to wash your hands and face.	
• Change your gown.	• Stroke your face, hair, or other parts of your body if you find that helps.
• Suck ice chips or sip water to keep your mouth moist.	• Offer ice chips and apply a cool cloth to your brow.
• Tell your support person or doctor, midwife, or nurse if you have the urge to push.	• Help you to do transition breathing (pant-pant-blow) to avoid pushing until the doctor, midwife, or nurse comes.

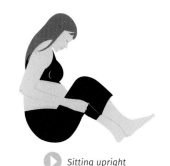

▶ *Sitting upright*

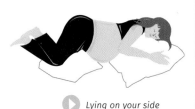

▶ *Lying on your side*

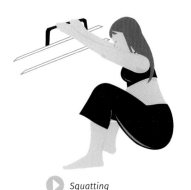

▶ *Squatting*

Body positions during labour and birth

Your body position can make labour easier. You should feel free to labour in any position that makes the process easier and to change positions as often as you want. Changing your position frequently during labour can promote the progress of your labour and help bring the baby down into the birth canal.

Sitting upright

Sitting up and reclining slightly is the most common position. This position may help your uterus to contract and may shorten the second stage of labour. The sitting position is a good position for the baby and also seems to help the baby move down the birth canal.

Lying on your side

Side lying is a comfortable position for labour and during birth. If you have certain heart conditions, hip joint problems, or varicose veins in your legs, this position may be easier and safer during birthing. If you choose this position, your labour coach can help to support your upper leg during the birth.

Squatting

The squatting position has two benefits. First, it makes bearing down (pushing) easier because gravity helps the uterus fall forward. This helps your baby move down the birth canal. Second, studies show that squatting helps widen the pelvis, giving the baby more room to move down and out. Some hospitals provide squatting bars on their birthing beds to help women who want to use this position.

Kneeling on all fours

This position often provides relief of back pain in labour. Some experts believe it may help a baby turn around into the proper position for birth if the baby has not done so on his own. Many women rock back and forth on all fours during contractions to help reduce their backache.

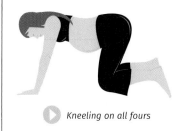

Kneeling on all fours

Hydrotherapy

Hydrotherapy involves the use of water during the first stage of labour as a pain and stress reliever.

Many women in labour find comfort in showers, whirlpool baths, and tub baths. Although hydrotherapy does not appear to shorten labour, when you feel less stressed, your body produces more "feel-good" hormones called *endorphins*. As well, lower stress levels during labour will enable the levels of the hormone oxytocin to rise. This helps to make contractions stronger and more regular.

Before you begin water therapy, it is best to get help from your nurse, midwife, or other support person. Water that is too hot can open (dilate) the blood vessels close to your skin and make your blood pressure drop. This may make you feel dizzy.

If you spend a long time in the tub, you must drink fluids or suck on ice chips so that your body does not become too dry (dehydrated). During water therapy, your baby's heart rate will still need to be counted at regular intervals (see page 151 "Monitoring your baby during labour") by your nurse or midwife. While you are in the tub, you and your labour coach can try some of the other techniques that make labour easier, such as massage, visualization, and special breathing.

Using your voice during labour

You may worry about crying out loudly during labour. Some women do, and others do not. Nurses, doctors, and midwives have heard women in labour making all kinds of sounds and noises. Many women vocalize during labour, others chant, moan, rock their bodies or heads from side to side, or cry out. These are all normal ways to cope with labour. You should never feel embarrassed about using your voice during labour.

Transcutaneous electric nerve stimulation (TENS)

TENS is a safe way to manage pain. It does not use medicines. It sends small electrical impulses through electrodes placed on your belly or back to the nerves under your skin. TENS is thought to work in two different ways:

- The electrical impulses block pain signals from going to the brain. For a woman in labour, the contractions may be causing pain, but your brain will not sense the pain.
- TENS triggers your body to release more of the body's feel-good hormone (endorphins).

If this method appeals to you, the hospital or birthing centre may be able to arrange for TENS treatments and will often rent the machines to you. You should contact them before your labour or speak with your health care provider about using TENS during one of your prenatal visits. These small devices can also be purchased from physical therapists or medical equipment stores. Check with your health insurance to see if this is covered.

Using medication for pain relief

Two main types of medicines are used to control pain during labour: painkillers and freezing.

- Painkillers are also known as analgesics. They dull the overall pain but do not make you lose all feeling in any part of your body.
- Freezing medicines are called local anaesthetics. They cause a loss of pain sensation and feeling in a specific parts of your body.

We suggest you talk to your health care team about the kind of pain relief you would like in your birth plan.

Painkillers (analgesics)

The most powerful painkillers are narcotics. You may be offered narcotics such as morphine during labour. They are usually given by injection into the muscles of the hip or sometimes through an intravenous (IV) line. They dull the pain and make you feel sleepy so that you can rest between contractions. They may also temporarily affect your baby because they can cross through the placenta.

Narcotics are usually given only in the early and active stages of your labour to make sure there is time for the effects to wear off before the baby is born. This helps to ensure your baby will be born alert and active. If you need pain medicine and your baby is born "sleepy," the doctors and nurses can safely give her a medicine that will wake her up quickly so she is able to breathe on her own.

Freezing (anaesthetics)

An *epidural* is a common type of local anaesthetic that blocks the pain of labour and birth. A doctor trained in this technique will insert a needle into a small space between the bones of your spine (vertebrae) and will inject the medicine. This numbs the nerves in that part of your body and blocks the pain.

When the doctor puts the medicine into your lower spine the first time, she will leave behind a small plastic tube (catheter) which will then be taped to the outside of your body. With this tube in place, you can receive more medication later.

Epidural medicine is often connected to a pump that provides you with a steady dose of the medication during labour. If you think you might want an epidural, discuss this with your health care provider before you go into labour. If you would like an epidural and your birth is taking place at home or at a birthing centre, the epidural would need to be administered in a hospital.

Nitrous oxide

Nitrous oxide is an anaesthetic gas given through a face mask. You hold the mask and start breathing in the gas just before a contraction begins. It will give you some pain relief within two or three breaths. The effects will go away about 5 minutes after you stop breathing the gas. Nitrous oxide is very safe and does not affect your baby.

The second stage of labour

The cervix is now open 10 centimetres and is fully dilated. The baby is ready to move down the birth canal. During the second stage of labour, contractions usually slow down. They happen 2 to 5 minutes apart and last about 45 to 90 seconds. This gives your body a much-needed rest between contractions.

Pushing

Most women feel an urge to push when their baby reaches a certain point in their pelvis. Pushing offers some relief from the pressure of labour. Pushing through a contraction has been described as a powerful release of stored energy that comes from deep within a woman's body and mind. You may feel powerful, strong, and in control when you begin to push.

When not to push

A couple of situations will delay pushing:

- If your cervix has not yet opened to 10 centimetres
- If your baby has not quite settled into the best position for pushing

Sometimes, the urge to push is so strong you simply cannot resist. With your nurse, midwife, or support person at your side to help you, you may be asked to put your knees very close to your chest and to use the pant-pant-blow method of special breathing until your cervix is fully open.

No urge to push

Some women do not feel the urge to push. They may need extra help and coaching to push their baby out. This may be the case for women who have had an epidural.

Some women go through a short time when they do not have any contractions or their contractions are very light and they have no urge to push.

If your cervix is fully dilated, but you do not feel an urge to push—relax and rest for a bit. The urge will come in time. Sometimes, epidurals can affect a woman's ability to push or can reduce the urge to push. Your nurse, doctor, or midwife will give you support and advice.

The natural rhythm of pushing

There is no right or wrong way to push. Although women are often encouraged to "take in a deep breath, hold it, and give one long steady hard push," this may not be the best method.

When women push naturally (without any instructions and based on their own rhythm), they tend to do three to five short pushes during each contraction. As the second stage of labour moves along, the number of pushes per contraction tends to increase. With natural pushing, women take in several big breaths of air with each pushing effort and slowly blow all the air out of their lungs. The natural way of pushing allows the most oxygen to reach your baby during the second stage of labour. Sometimes this natural way of pushing may take a few minutes longer, but it is less tiring.

Making room for the birth

Often, a baby is born with little or no tearing of the perineum (the skin at the bottom of the vagina). The health care provider may massage the skin around the perineum, helping it to stretch. About 70% of first-time mothers will need some kind of small and simple repair to their perineum after childbirth. While the tears are repaired, the doctor may freeze the area with a local anaesthetic to make you more comfortable.

Research has shown that such small tears heal better, with less pain, than a larger cut called an **episiotomy.** An episiotomy is a cut about 2.5 to 5 cm (1 to 2 in) long. It is made at the bottom of your vagina toward the rectum or off to one side. Before making the cut, your health care provider will freeze that part of your body with a local anaesthetic.

In some cases, an episiotomy is done to make more room for the baby's head and shoulders or if it is important to speed up the birth because of concern for the baby. An episiotomy should be done only if needed.

The third stage of labour

This stage of labour begins after the baby has been born and ends when the placenta separates from the uterus and comes out of your uterus (about 30 minutes after the birth). Other than having a few mild contractions to push out your placenta, your work is done, and this is a time of relief.

As long as your uterus shrinks and stays firm (and there is no unusual bleeding), it is best to watch and wait for the delivery of the placenta.

If you need any repairs to your skin from tearing or an episiotomy, these repairs will be done after you have delivered the placenta. Finally, to help your uterus shrink and to minimize the bleeding, your health care provider is likely to give you an injection or IV infusion of oxytocin, a synthetic hormone. This reduces the amount of blood that a woman may lose after birth and can prevent too much bleeding (postpartum hemorrhage).

THE THIRD STAGE OF LABOUR

You can:

- *Take a moment to relax.*

- *Hold your baby skin-to-skin on your bare chest.*

- *Ask for a warmed blanket if you are shaky or chilled.*

- *Push out the placenta when it is ready to come out.*

Your support person can:

- *Relax and enjoy the moment with you.*

- *Bond with the baby. He or she can provide skin-to-skin contact if you are unable.*

- *Help you get into a comfortable position to breastfeed.*

- *Offer you something to drink and wipe your face and hands with a damp cloth.*

People to call after the baby arrives

During this time, your nurse or midwife will feel the size and shape of your uterus to make sure that it continues to shrink and that the bleeding slows down. Both you and the nurse or midwife will be caring for your baby during this stage. If you and your baby are medically stable, your baby should be placed on his or her tummy, skin-to-skin on your bare chest. This skin-to-skin time should be uninterrupted and unhurried. Your baby may root and begin to breastfeed. Skin-to-skin contact is important for all mothers and babies regardless of the mother's infant-feeding decision.

You may tremble, feel chilly, or even feel like you may throw up (have nausea). The nausea should pass quickly and a warmed blanket will soothe your chills.

After the birth

Once born, your baby will be placed skin-to-skin and needs to have the umbilical cord clamped and cut. Your midwife or nurse will help to dry your baby. At the same time, they will make sure that your baby has started to breathe properly and will observe the baby's colour, tone, and do an Apgar score based on these. For more information on Apgar score see page 168.

Cord blood gases

Immediately after birth, a "cord blood gases" test may be done. The health care provider will take a sample of blood from a section of the umbilical cord after it has been cut; this is to check the oxygen and pH levels. The pH level measures the balance of chemicals in the baby's blood and is an important way to learn about the baby's well-being at birth.

The fourth stage of labour

The fourth stage of labour begins after the placenta is out and lasts about 2 hours. It is a time to rest, enjoy, and recover. During this time, you will be watched closely as you rest after the birth. Your nurse or midwife will check your blood pressure, heart rate, breathing, the position of the top of your uterus, and the amount of bleeding from your vagina. Those tests can be done with baby skin-to-skin as long as both the mother and baby are medically stable. Other procedures, such as measuring and weighing the baby, should be delayed until after the first feeding.

Bonding with your baby

You and your baby should be together after the birth. The best place for your baby is naked on your bare chest or abdomen for at least the first hour after birth and until after the first breastfeed so that you have skin-to-skin contact. This will make it easier for your baby to "latch"—the way in which baby attaches to the breast for feeding. Skin-to-skin contact is important no matter the feeding decision. Health care staff members understand the bonding process and will support you to do this. They will dim the lights so it will be easier for the baby to open his or her eyes.

Skin-to-skin contact is the best way to bond with your baby and to keep your baby warm and comfortable right after birth. Talk quietly and softly using your normal tone of voice. You may notice your baby's face turning toward the sound of your voice and his or her eyes searching to make contact with yours.

For the first hour or two after the birth, you will both be very alert. This is the best time for both bonding and the first breastfeeding.

Newborn screening tests

All newborns are tested and screened to make sure they are healthy. Blood samples are taken in the first few days of life to test for disorders that can be present in a baby that seems to be healthy. All Canadian newborns are screened for conditions that affect how they digest food, how they produce hormones (which can affect normal growth and development), and for cystic fibrosis. The results will be sent to your health care provider. You will learn of the results only if there is a concern.

Screening for hearing may be done while you are in the hospital or later when your baby visits his or her health care provider. If you are not in the hospital, your midwife will arrange to have these tests done. If a hearing problem is found, a further test will be needed. Hearing problems can affect your baby's language and social skills.

Over the next few days, use every chance you get to talk to your baby. Hold your baby close and continue to have as much skin-to-skin contact as you can. Handle your newborn slowly and carefully. Support the baby's head and neck and feed your baby whenever he is hungry.

Apgar score

A simple and quick method of assessing newborn health is done 1 minute after the birth and again 5 minutes later. The Apgar score is essential to help health care providers know whether your baby will need any special care. Five areas are rated during an Apgar score test, including the baby's:

1. Heart rate
2. Breathing
3. Muscle tone
4. Reflexes
5. Skin colour

Each of these areas is measured and—depending on how the baby responds—rated from 0 to 2. Zero is the poorest response, and 2 is the best response. The total number of this test is the Apgar score. Most babies score between 7 and 10.

An example follows:

A baby is born with a heart rate of 140 (scores 2), has a good strong cry (scores 2), with some movements (scores 1), coughing (scores 2), and pink all over (scores 2). The total Apgar score, in this case, will be 9.

Any score over 7 at 5 minutes after birth predicts a healthy baby.

Apgar scores			
	Score 0	*Score 1*	*Score 2*
Heart rate	Absent	Slow (< 100 per minute)	> 100 per minute
Breathing	Absent	Weak	Good, strong cry
Muscle tone	Limp	Some movement	Active movements
Reflexes	No response	Grimace, whimpering	Cough or sneeze
Skin colour	Blue or pale	Body pink, arms and legs blue	Completely pink

Medical help during labour and birth

Induction of labour

An overdue baby is only one reason for inducing labour. If your water breaks without labour starting on its own, you and your doctor or midwife will have to decide between inducing labour and waiting for it to start on its own. Either choice may be the correct one. It all depends on factors such as how long the membranes have been ruptured, whether the cervix is ripe, the risk of infection, and your own feelings.

There are other reasons why it may be best to induce labour at 40 weeks of pregnancy or before:

- If the pregnant woman has high blood pressure that is getting worse
- If the pregnant woman has an illness such as diabetes
- If there are signs that the baby is not growing well
- If there are other medical concerns

Labour should be induced only for these valid medical reasons.

How labour is induced

There are several common ways to induce labour.

Ripen the cervix: Normally, the cervix begins to get softer, wider, and shorter before labour starts. This is called *ripening.* If your cervix is not getting ready for labour on its own, and you are having labour induced, your health care provider may try to ripen your cervix. The most common way to do this is by placing a special gel or insert that contains a certain hormone (prostaglandin E2) onto your cervix or your vagina. Another way your health care provider can gently ripen your cervix is by placing a rubber tube with a balloon on the end into the cervix and then blowing up the balloon. It is important to soften or ripen the cervix before inducing labour.

Rupture the membranes: If the membranes of the amniotic sac are still in place, the next step may be to break them. This is done using a simple method: a specialized instrument is inserted into the cervix to puncture the membrane. The procedure feels similar to a routine examination of your vagina. For most women, labour will begin within 12 hours after the membranes are ruptured. This is most likely to happen if the cervix is also ripe. Some women have their membranes ruptured in order to speed up labour that has already started on its own.

Start the contractions: To bring about contractions of the uterus, your health care provider can give you a drug called *oxytocin,* which is almost the same as the natural hormone you would produce. It is given by IV, and it is recommended to start continuous monitoring of your baby's heart rate.

How long does induction of labour take? The process of induction may take several days, especially if cervical ripening is required.

Breech babies

Most babies are born head first. During the last month of pregnancy, they lie with their heads towards the birth canal. A baby is in a **breech position** when the baby's rear end is facing the birth canal.

If you are near your due date (the last 4 to 6 weeks) and your health care provider suspects a breech baby, an ultrasound will be done to confirm the position, size, and health of your baby.

If the ultrasound confirms a breech position, you will need to discuss the choices for the best birth. For some breech babies, the way their legs or head are sitting in the uterus will mean that a caesarean birth is safest. Other breech babies can be safely born through the vagina, as long as certain conditions are in place. You would need to discuss this with your health care provider. A third option is to turn the baby to a head down position, using a technique called *external cephalic version (ECV)*. After you have all the information you need and are aware of all the options available to you, you may choose to have the ECV, a normal vaginal breech birth, or a planned caesarean birth. Your health care provider will present options that are safe and available for your particular situation and help you choose the safest way of birthing your baby.

Assisted births: forceps or vacuum extraction

Sometimes, a baby needs to be helped out of the birth canal. A health care provider may choose to assist the birth using **forceps** or a **vacuum extraction.** These methods are used when the second stage of labour has lasted a very long time, the mother is tired and is having a hard time pushing, but the baby is low enough to be born through the vagina with a little help. An assisted birth is also often used when a baby's heartbeat is showing signs of distress.

Both forceps and vacuum extractor methods are common and safe in experienced hands. You may require additional pain medication, and there may be an increased risk of a vaginal tear or the need for an episiotomy.

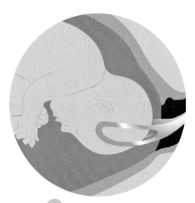

Forceps assistance

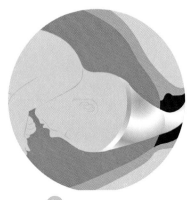

Vacuum extraction

- **Forceps** are two slim, curved instruments that can slide around the baby's head inside the birth canal. Once they are in place, the doctor can adjust the position of the baby's head and help the woman to bring the baby down and out.
- The **vacuum method** is also called a *suction-assisted birth*. It involves placing a plastic cup that is held in place by suction on top of the baby's head. A handle is attached to the cup. This allows the health care provider to gently assist the baby's birth.

Caesarean births

A **caesarean birth** (also called a *caesarean section* or a *C-section*) is an operation that opens the pregnant woman's abdomen to remove the baby from the uterus. In Canada, about one-quarter of women have caesarean births. Sometimes, for medical reasons, this surgery is planned in advance and done before labour begins. At other times, if problems arise for the mother or the baby during labour, it is done when labour is already in progress.

The most common reason for a caesarean birth is when labour is not progressing as would be expected. Despite good and regular contractions, the cervix stops dilating for several hours or the baby does not move down into the pelvis for birth. In these cases, and when all else has been tried without success, a caesarean birth becomes necessary.

Concern about the baby's well-being is the second most common reason for a caesarean birth. This happens most often when there are unusual changes in the baby's heart rate during labour. In some cases, this may be confirmed with a fetal scalp blood sample. If the health care team strongly suspects that the baby may not be tolerating labour, and if the birth is not about to happen soon, a caesarean birth will be considered.

The third most common reason for a caesarean birth is the mother's history of having a caesarean birth in the past.

If you had a caesarean birth before, you should be aware that you have an excellent chance of having a vaginal birth and that this is a safe option. Some women may not want to try labour again because they are afraid of having a long painful labour that will only end in another caesarean birth. If this is how you feel, talk to your health care provider.

Other less common reasons for caesarean births include the following:

- The baby is in a breech position (see page 170).
- There is bleeding from a separated placenta.
- There is bleeding from a placenta that covers the cervix (also known as *placenta previa*).

Sometimes a caesarean birth is needed for the mother's health, as in the case of serious illness such as toxemia or severe cases of diabetes. If a mother has an active herpes infection or untreated HIV or high viral loads of HIV, the baby will be born by caesarean birth to prevent the disease from spreading to the baby during the birth.

Childbirth is unpredictable. No one can fully control it, no matter how prepared she is. Whether you give birth vaginally or by caesarean, the goal of pregnancy is for you to become the mother of a healthy child. How you get to that goal is not as important as the goal itself. All women should be aware that a caesarean birth may be necessary. When you create your birth plan, make sure you include what you would like to do if you need to have a caesarean birth. You can still breastfeed if you've had a caesarean birth.

If you give birth at a free-standing birthing centre or at home, you would need to be transferred to a hospital if you request an epidural for labour pain, have medical problems, excessive bleeding, or need a procedure such as a caesarean birth.

Postpartum hemorrhage

All mothers experience some bleeding after the birth, but 7% to 10% have postpartum hemorrhage, which is excessive bleeding. This is more common if the baby was large, if the labour was long and difficult, or if it was a multiple birth (twins or more). In the past, many women died of this bleeding, but with modern medical care, postpartum hemorrhage is usually easy to treat.

How to prevent postpartum hemorrhage

Breastfeeding and massage of a soft uterus are effective ways of preventing excessive postpartum bleeding, because both stimulate the uterus to contract.

Recent studies also show that giving women a hormone-like medicine (oxytocin) can prevent the risk of postpartum hemorrhage by up to 40%. Most hospitals now give this medicine to all women in labour, during either the second or third stage of labour. It is given by injection into a muscle or by intravenous line. Midwives can also give oxytocin at home or during birth centre births.

How long will you stay in hospital or birthing centre?

Benefits of going home early

If you give birth in a hospital or birthing centre, you may go home as early as a day or two after your baby's birth when you and your baby are medically stable.

Prenatal classes will have covered the information that you will need when you first go home with your baby. Nurses and midwives are experts in teaching new mothers how to care for newborn babies. They will help with breastfeeding and help to make sure baby is attaching (latching) well to the breast to feed. Many hospitals offer classes to parents before they leave to go home. Ask questions. Do not be shy about calling the contact numbers they will provide you with if you have questions once you get home. In many centers, breastfeeding classes are available to take during pregnancy. These classes are usually offered by a registered nurse who is skilled with helping breastfeeding mothers or an International Board Certified Lactation Consultant.

Follow-up home care

In Canada, we have a public health system that provides follow-up home care after birth. This level of follow-up care varies from province to province. If you are going home early, it is very important that you have an early follow-up for the baby. Some hospitals have a discharge class that parents have to attend before they go home. Some hospitals or health regions have a care plan for women and their babies after birth. This can range from telephone follow-ups, visits to clinics, breastfeeding clinics, and home visits, depending on your needs and your baby's need and what services are available in your area.

The Society of Obstetricians and Gynaecologists of Canada and the Canadian Paediatric Society have issued a combined statement about how to know when it is safe for mothers and babies to leave the hospital. They clearly state that early home follow-up is essential to early discharge. By having a follow-up at home, you can be sure that feeding is well established, that the baby is getting enough breast milk in his first days, and that jaundice is not a problem. Getting help early is important if your baby has any of these problems.

An International Board Certified Lactation Consultant (IBCLC) is a person who has received extensive training to help mothers during pregnancy and after giving birth with challenging breastfeeding problems. If you feel that you need help from an IBCLC, talk to your health care provider and ask for a referral or check with the Canadian Lactation Consultant Association at www.clca-accl.ca and International Lactation Consultant Association at www.ilca.org/why-ibclc/falc.

FOLLOW-UP HOME CARE INFORMATION

Phone number for public health clinic, hospital, or helpline:

_____

Date and time of first visit:

_____

Date and time of second visit:

_____

Nurse or midwife's name:

_____

Things I need to ask the nurse or midwife during my home visit:

1. _____
2. _____
3. _____
4. _____
5. _____
6. _____
7. _____
8. _____
9. _____
10. _____

If home visits are available in your area, the nurse or midwife will examine you and your baby and answer your questions about caring for yourself and your newborn. The visit usually includes time to talk about your body, breastfeeding, diapering, and baths, bonding with your baby, having sex again, and birth control. This private and close care will help give you the confidence you need to look after your new baby. It is a good idea to write your questions down before the nurse or midwife arrives so that you will remember what you wanted to ask (see the sidebar called "Follow-up home care information").

Longer hospital stays

Sometimes, it's best to stay in the hospital a little longer than usual. This may be the case if there were problems during the birth, if you had a long labour or a caesarean birth, or if you or your baby needs special attention or care. As well, a longer hospital stay may be important if your hospital does not offer a home care program or if you do not have enough support at home. Talk to your maternity nurse, midwife, or doctor if you have concerns about going home.

If your baby is unwell or not able to breastfeed at birth for medical reasons, you should talk to the health care staff about how to express your own milk and save it for when your baby is well enough to feed. This can be done by hand—called *hand expression*—or using a pump. Be sure to talk to a health care provider so that you select a breast pump that is best suited for your needs.

If things do not happen as you planned . . .

Despite modern medicine, babies are sometimes born with a serious illness or with problems the health care team did not expect. It is very rare for babies to die. All parents hope for the best during pregnancy, and most have bonded deeply with their unborn child before the birth. They begin to think of their baby as a person, as the newest member of their family.

It is a great shock when a baby is born with an illness, with genetic or physical differences, or without signs of life. Some mothers might feel their bodies have betrayed them. Everyone copes with such a sad loss differently, experiencing a range of different emotions. Some worry that they may have done something to make it happen. This is almost never true.

Parents can feel a deep sense of disappointment even if the baby is born alive but with a serious illness or health problem. They feel grief because the child they imagined all through pregnancy does not exist. In some cases, it might take a while to adjust to a new baby with health problems. It may take time before all the challenges are discovered. There are many resources, both in the hospital and in the community, to help mothers and families adjust to life with a baby who has special medical or other needs.

Saying goodbye to a baby

The deepest and most profound sense of loss comes from the death of a baby. Whether the death happens early in the pregnancy, is detected later in pregnancy, or happens after birth, the loss causes a range of emotions such as intense sadness, shock, disbelief, and even anger. Because bonding often occurs long before a baby is born, many parents have trouble coping with their loss. It is unthinkable to imagine life without the baby you longed for, had hopes and dreams for, and in many cases, planned your life around. How does life go on?

For parents and family, the grieving process is a necessary part of healing. Grieving helps parents cope—but no two people grieve

YOU AND YOUR PARTNER— SHARING THE LOSS

You may find that your relationship with your partner is strained following a loss. You may find it difficult to talk and communicate effectively with each other. Normal, everyday tasks may be difficult to complete, and you may find it hard to connect on both emotional and physical levels. Feeling anger toward your partner or others is a common reaction as you try to cope. It is normal to feel this way.

Be patient with each other. Tell each other how you are feeling and be as open and honest as you can. Seek professional counselling. If your partner can't talk about the baby's death right now, remind yourself that you will be able to talk to each other about it in the future. Your baby is not forgotten. Everyone deals with grief in his or her way and at his or her own pace. Make an extra effort to be tender and kind toward each other.

the same way. All parents can benefit from grief or bereavement support at such a tragic time in their lives.

Although every hospital will have its own supports to help cope with pregnancy and infant loss, your health care team will be able to guide you through the process of saying goodbye. Here are some things you should expect:

- To be given the opportunity to see and hold your baby (if the baby died because of birth defects, some parents may be afraid to do this, but in almost all cases, what the parents imagine is worse than it really is)
- To be given the opportunity to collect momentos and create positive memories (pictures, hand and footprints or moulds, a lock of hair, naming ceremony, etc.)
- To not be rushed
- To be given privacy
- To be treated with respect and dignity (especially in cases of early loss)
- To be provided with resources about funeral planning and memorial services
- To be given the opportunity to talk about your feelings
- To be provided with resources that link grieving families to services offered in the community. (Visit the Pregnancy and Infant Loss Network (PAIL) website at www.pailnetwork.ca or call 1-888-301-7276.)

You may feel very alone, but there is a great deal of support available to you.

My baby's journal

_____
_____
_____
_____
_____
_____
_____
_____
_____
_____
_____
_____
_____
_____
_____
_____
_____
_____
_____
_____
_____
_____

BABY'S BIRTHDAY

Date:

Time of birth:

Weight:

Length:

Hair:

Eye colour:

Health care providers:

Notes:

My to-do list

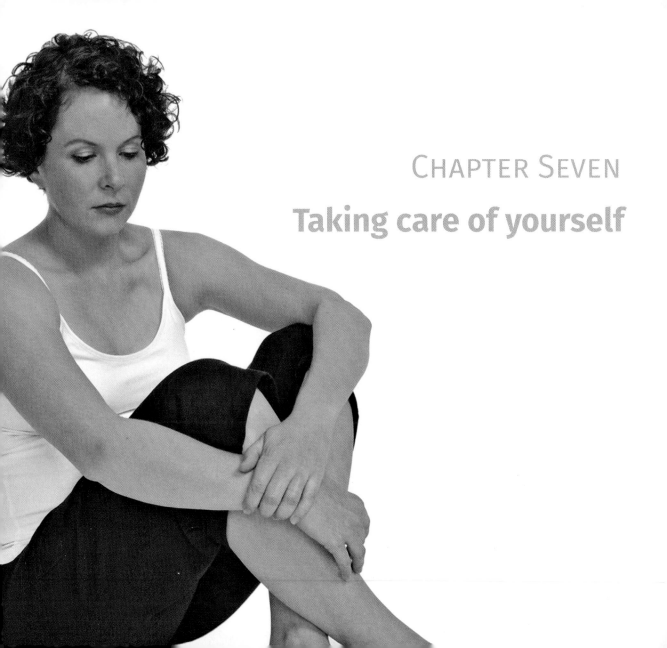

CHAPTER SEVEN

Taking care of yourself

RECIPE FOR REST

Many mothers have a burst of energy right after their babies are born and then feel very tired. They will need to watch their baby for hunger cues and their baby will need to feed eight times or more in 24 hours. Babies need to feed both during the day and night. Regular feedings and caring for a newborn require a great deal of energy, so it is important to do what you can to be healthy and to look after your needs now and after you give birth.

HERE IS AN EASY RECIPE TO REMEMBER:

R **Relax** whenever you can. Take a nap, read, watch television, and **sleep when the baby sleeps!**

E **Eat healthily and drink when you feel thirsty.**

S **Share** the responsibility of your new baby with your partner, family, and friends. Ask for help.

T **Take time** to enjoy the baby. Ask for help with housework and other chores.

Welcome to the chapter about you. Yes, about you. One of the most important things you can do for your new baby is to take care of yourself. Looking after a newborn is much easier if you are well-rested and healthy. Your body has just been through many months of change.

You should know that you will need some time to get your body back to where it was before your pregnancy. And you'll also be making some emotional adjustments—to the new member of your family and to the hormonal changes that come after birth.

Plan to see your health care provider within 6 weeks after the birth to make sure that your body has healed well. You may have heard about the "baby blues." There is a section on the subject. You may also have heard about "postpartum depression," which is different. This chapter will also cover common questions about discomforts after birth, when the bleeding after the birth should stop, when to expect your periods to return, and different birth control options.

You will need time to get used to all the changes that come with having a baby. Now is a good time to ask for help from family and friends and to accept their offers to cook meals, clean the house, do laundry, or babysit your other children. Taking care of yourself is important.

Your changing body after the birth

The many changes your body went through during pregnancy happened slowly over 9 months. It will take about the same amount of time for things to return to normal, so be patient with yourself.

After the birth of your baby, you can feel your uterus if you press on your lower belly (just a little above your pubic bone). Six weeks after birth, your uterus will be almost its normal size, and you will not be able to feel it any more by pressing on your belly. Breastfeeding helps the uterus shrink back to its normal size more quickly.

The area between your rectum and your vagina is called your **perineum.** It stretched during the baby's birth. It may feel swollen, bruised, and tender. You may have stitches from a tear or an episiotomy. These stitches will dissolve over time, but they can be itchy while they heal. Keep doing your Kegel exercises (see page 59). They will help the stretched muscles in your perineum regain their tone. Some women feel numbness in their perineum. This goes away over time. You may also experience some urinary incontinence, which will usually go away with time and Kegel exercises.

The baby blues

After giving birth, it is normal to cry for no reason, to feel anxious, frightened, and sad. More than 70% of new mothers feel a little depressed after birth. For most women, this happens within a couple of days of the birth. You may have heard it called "the baby blues." It may be linked to the changing levels of pregnancy hormones and may also come from feelings of loss, because the baby is no longer inside you. These feelings may last for hours or days. For most women, they go away within 2 weeks without any treatment.

You may feel a wide range of changing emotions. One minute you might feel happy, the next minute sad. You may feel very tired and then get a burst of energy. You may have trouble sleeping or making decisions. You may feel confident then insecure. You may feel as though you will never get your old life or body back. You may not be interested in sex at all. All these feelings are completely normal. Now is when you reach out to your partner, family, and friends for support.

THE SIGNS OF POSTPARTUM DEPRESSION

- *My baby blues have not gone away after 2 weeks.*
- *I don't feel like my usual self.*
- *I have strong feelings of sadness or guilt.*
- *I often feel very anxious or worried.*
- *I have strong feelings of hopelessness or helplessness.*
- *I cannot sleep, even when I am tired.*
- *I sleep all the time, even when my baby is awake.*
- *I cannot eat, even when I am hungry.*
- *I cannot eat because I am never hungry or because I feel sick.*
- *I worry about the baby too much; I'm obsessed with the baby.*
- *I do not worry about the baby at all; it's almost like I don't care.*
- *I am having anxiety or panic attacks.*
- *I feel angry toward the baby.*
- *I think about hurting my baby or myself.*

(Continued)

The signs of postpartum depression (Continued)

*If you have any of these signs, talk to your health care provider. If you know a new mother who has these signs, get help for her. Counselling and treatment will help the feelings go away. Do not wait for things to get better. Call your health care provider or your local crisis intervention line **right away.***

Perinatal mental health

If the baby blues seem to be getting worse instead of better, or if they last more than 2 weeks, you may be moving into postpartum depression. This happens to approximately 20% of new mothers. Some signs will alert you to seek help—and help is available.

You may feel sad or have a sense of hopelessness. You may feel angry about "being on call 24/7." You may wonder if you are able to look after the baby and feel someone else would do a better job or feel frustrated or even angry when your baby cries. Thoughts or pictures may jump into your head about harming your baby or yourself. If you have any of these feelings—***seek help immediately.***

Postpartum depression is a clinical problem. It is not your fault. There is help for you and your family. Talk to your health care provider about services for women and their families dealing with mental health issues. Effective and safe treatments can include therapy and medication. Most medications suggested are safe for your baby when you are breastfeeding. Getting prompt treatment will help you to feel better and improve the health of your baby.

Anxiety and depression can go from the normal feelings that any new parent may experience to an overwhelming problem. If you or your partner are suffering with anxiety or depression there is help available. Don't be afraid to ask.

Normal vaginal discharge

Be prepared for some bloody discharge from your vagina after birth. It's called lochia, and it is made up of blood and tissue from the lining of the uterus that your body will expel after birth. At first, the lochia is bright red and may contain a few small clots. Bright red blood may flow again for short periods during or after breastfeeding. This is because breastfeeding causes mild contractions in the uterus, helping to get rid of the lining. Also, blood may collect in the vagina while you are lying down and can gush out for a short time when you stand up. This is normal for the first few days.

Within a few days, your flow will begin to decrease and will become darker. As this happens, it is normal to notice some bloody spotting. Eventually, your flow will turn whitish or yellowish and will slowly stop. This can last from 10 days to 5 weeks. If you have given birth before, your flow may not be the same as it was with your last baby. It is best to use sanitary pads during this time, not tampons.

If your flow is heavier than you think is normal, is heavier than a period, or if it smells bad, check with your health care provider.

Having sex again

It is up to you to decide when you feel ready to have sex again after the birth. It's good to wait until you feel ready—at both the emotional and physical levels. Your body, mind, and spirit need time to adjust to the changes that childbirth and motherhood bring. If you are like most new mothers, you will likely be using all your energy to look after the baby. You may feel quite tired for the first few weeks.

Most couples do not have sex for 4 to 6 weeks after birth. It takes that long for your birth canal and uterus to resume their normal shape and size and for you to feel comfortable. There are profound changes in many hormones after pregnancy, and your sex drive may be quite low because of those changes. For some couples, the baby's demands make it hard to find the energy to have sex as often as before. Keep in mind that your partner has not been pregnant for

UNUSUAL BLEEDING AND VAGINAL DISCHARGE

*It's normal for the blood flow to slowly decrease with each passing day. If your flow has been decreasing, but suddenly becomes a lot heavier with bright red blood (which soaks through one or more maxi-pads within 2 hours and does not slow down or stop when you take time to rest), do not wait—**go to a hospital immediately**. If your flow has not fully stopped after 6 weeks, make an appointment to see your health care provider.*

The following are not normal:
- *Developing large blood clots*
- *Having unusual vaginal discharge*
- *Having a bad smell coming from your vagina*
- *Having a high fever*

If you notice any of these situations, you need to see your health care provider. He or she may suggest treatment to deal with these issues.

9 months and may not be as aware of your physical (and emotional) condition as you are. So, you will both have to adjust to the changes a baby brings, which means talking—about your feelings (and frustrations, too).

You may simply feel worn out by late-night feedings, all the excitement, and the added responsibility. You may also feel mildly depressed and not be interested in sex (part of the "baby blues"). Some new mothers feel insecure and do not like their body image and may not feel attractive for the first little while. All these feelings and worries are normal. It may take a few weeks or several months before your sex drive returns. If you have any concerns about starting to have sex again with your partner, make an appointment with your health care provider for a check-up.

Once you are ready to have sex again, it is important to think about what type of birth control is best for you at this time. (See pages 190 to 194 for more information about birth control.) You **can** get pregnant . . . again!

After childbirth, estrogen levels fall sharply, and this can result in many changes in your body, including vaginal dryness. If sexual intercourse is painful because of dryness, there are products available to help lubricate your vagina. They can be found at the drugstore in the same section where you can buy condoms. You can also try changing positions to see if one is more comfortable than another. If you feel discomfort for a long time, talk to your health care provider.

Common discomforts after giving birth

Tender breasts

Your body has been preparing for your baby to be born and to breastfeed ever since you became pregnant. The early milk in your breast is called *colostrum* and this is the milk that your baby first drinks. Colostrum provides special immune protection and also has the perfect combination of nutrients that your new baby needs to get off to a good start.

After your baby is born and your body makes new milk, it begins to mix with the colostrum. When this happens, day two to four after giving birth, many mothers notice that their breasts feel fuller, warmer, and a bit tender. Breastfeeding your baby at least eight times in 24 hours will help prevent your breasts from becoming too full. The stimulation of your baby sucking and drinking your milk also helps your body make more milk for your baby.

Wear a nursing bra or a comfortable bra that is supportive and does not have underwires or seams that dig in. Using cold compresses between feedings and warm compresses for 2 to 3 minutes just before feeding can also help you feel more comfortable. If your breasts become overly full, hard, and painful, see page 229 to learn more about engorgement.

Vaginal pain

It's normal for the perineum (the area around your anus and vagina) to be swollen, bruised, and tender after you have given birth. For some women, this soreness lasts up to 6 weeks. If you have stitches, you may feel even more discomfort. Most women are discharged from the hospital with instructions that they can use acetaminophen and/or ibuprofen for pain, which is safe to use when breastfeeding. If the pain persists, talk to your health care provider. See the sidebar for suggestions to help find relief from vaginal pain and swelling.

Cramping

Pains that feel like strong menstrual cramps are called ***after-pains.*** They are caused by the uterus shrinking. They may feel worse

You may find relief from vaginal pain and swelling by doing the following:

- *Apply ice packs to the perineal area for the first 24 hours. Ice packs and cold compresses should be removed after 10 to 20 minutes and be reapplied every hour as needed.*
- *Ice packs should be wrapped in a towel or facecloth and not applied directly to the skin.*
- *Women can use cold compresses, a bag of ice or of frozen veggies, or a frozen water-soaked maxi-pad or baby diaper to place in their underwear.*
- *Rest as much as possible.*
- *Let the perineum "air-dry" while resting.*
- *Use a pillow or an inflatable ring when sitting. Inflatable rings are available at most drugstores.*
- *Soak the perineal area in warm water a few times a day and after bowel movements. A sitz bath filled with a few inches*
(Continued)

(Continued)

of water and placed on the toilet seat is convenient. Sitz baths can be purchased at the drugstore or home health store. If you are using your bathtub for perineal soaks, have it cleaned first and ensure that someone is present to help you in and out of the tub for the first few times.

- *Take pain medications recommended by your health care provider.*

during breastfeeding. First-time mothers may not feel after-pains. Try taking a warm bath or put a heating pad across your belly. You can use the medication that was recommended by your health care provider. If that is not helping, contact your health care provider. The deep breathing and relaxation techniques you learned during pregnancy may also help.

Bowel movements

You may not have a bowel movement for 2 to 3 days after the birth of your baby. The muscles in your abdomen that help you have a bowel movement have become stretched and do not work as well. Also, if you have not eaten very much or if you had painkillers during or after giving birth, your bowels will be sluggish.

Do what you can to avoid hard stools. Drink plenty of fluids, and eat foods high in fibre, such as bran muffins, bran cereal, fresh fruit, and vegetables. Stool softeners made with psyllium or natural fibre (such as coarse ground flaxseed) can be bought at the drugstore.

Hemorrhoids

Grape-like swellings around the rectum are called *hemorrhoids*. They are often painful and itchy. During a difficult bowel movement, especially with a hard stool, they may ooze a little blood.

As with vaginal or perineum pain, you can help reduce the swelling by freezing a damp maxi-pad and then putting it in your underwear. Cool witch hazel compresses can also provide relief.

You may prefer to lie down, rather than sit. This will take the pressure off your bottom until the hemorrhoids heal. There are special creams, sprays, and ointments that help decrease hemorrhoid discomfort that can safely be used while breastfeeding. Talk to your pharmacist or health care provider about what might work for you.

Problems with urinating

Right after the birth or for the first day or so you may find it hard to urinate. This is most true if you had a long second stage, a catheter, or if you have stitches or a small tear in your vagina. To help the flow of urine get started, try turning on the taps in the bathroom sink so you can hear the water. To help take away the sting, urinate while taking a shower or a bath or try squeezing warm water from a bottle over that part of your body when you urinate.

Later, you may find you have to urinate quite often or that you have trouble knowing when the urine is going to start flowing. You may lose urine with a cough, sneeze, or when you exercise. This is called **urinary incontinence.** It happens when the pelvic floor muscles get stretched—as they do during pregnancy and childbirth. You can help strengthen your muscles by doing Kegel exercises (see page 59). For most women, this problem slowly goes away. Physiotherapists who specialize in pelvic health and urinary incontinence can check if you are doing Kegels correctly by using biofeedback or by checking with a finger in the vagina.

Your body shape after pregnancy

The muscles in your abdomen stretched a lot during your pregnancy. They will slowly tighten back into their pre-pregnancy shape. During pregnancy, you gained weight slowly and it may take a few months to lose that weight. Do not try to lose weight quickly by eating a low-calorie diet. It's far better to eat a range of healthy foods and to resume exercise and increase it slowly over time.

Walking at a good pace is an excellent toning exercise. Carry your baby in a sling or baby carrier or push your baby in a stroller or carriage and your baby will enjoy it, too. Walk briskly or do a similar exercise for at least 20 minutes a day to start getting back into shape. In some communities, you may be able to find postnatal fitness classes to meet your needs. Joining these classes will give you a chance to meet other new mothers and talk about the things that are on your mind. If you are short of sleep and find that meeting all of your baby's needs is stressful, talking to other mothers about their lives and sharing tips on how to cope will help. In many communities there are group activities or exercise classes for new mothers and their babies.

Not getting enough sleep and feeling stressed can raise the levels of a stress hormone called **cortisol.** This makes you store fat, especially around the middle. Getting enough sleep is vital to losing weight and is not easy for new parents.

Menstrual periods

Menstruation may not start again for several months or until you stop breastfeeding altogether. However, your ovaries may release an egg before your period returns. This means you could become pregnant again without having your period return. If you want to avoid pregnancy, you should begin using birth control as soon as you plan to be sexually active after the birth (usually 4 to 6 weeks).

If you are not breastfeeding, your menstrual period will probably start again 4 to 9 weeks after the birth. Your period may be longer, shorter, heavier, or lighter than before pregnancy. It will likely return to what is normal for you after a few cycles.

Birth control choices

If you do not want to get pregnant again right away, you and your partner should decide what type of birth control is best for you now. You **can** get pregnant even if your menstrual periods have not started again yet. It is important to decide which birth control method is right for you and your partner and to have it ready before you begin having sex again. Talk to your health care provider about your choices.

Lactation amenorrhea method/LAM: This is a natural method of short term birth control that is 98% effective if **ALL** of the following conditions are met:

- You are exclusively breastfeeding, meaning that you feed your baby only breastmilk.
- Your period has not started since the birth of your baby.
- Your baby is less than 6 months old.

The pill, the patch, and the ring are hormonal contraceptives that work in a similar manner and must be prescribed by a health care provider. The pill is taken orally (by mouth), the patch is applied to the skin, and the ring is inserted vaginally.

If you are not breastfeeding, you can begin using the pill, the patch, or the ring 3 to 4 weeks after your child is born. However, breastfeeding mothers who wish to use hormonal contraceptives, should use a birth control pill that is less likely to decrease milk production. The progestin-only type pill (mini-pill) does not appear to affect breastfeeding in most women.

If you are breastfeeding and wish to start hormonal birth control, you will have to wait at least 6 weeks after your baby is born before you begin. It will be important that if you do so, your breastfeeding is going well and your baby is gaining her proper weight. Consider starting with the mini-pill before switching to a longer acting form of hormonal contraceptive like the patch or the shot because it is easier to switch from the mini-pill to a different birth control method if your milk supply is affected.

Injectable contraceptives (the shot): This is also a hormonal-type contraceptive. A health care provider will give you an injection once every 3 months. This form of birth control is safe, easy, and not too costly. You may start this method immediately after giving birth if you are not breastfeeding. Otherwise, you may begin using it 6 weeks after your child is born. Talk to your health care provider to learn more.

Intrauterine device (IUD): You can be fitted with an IUD by your health care provider 4 weeks after birth or it can also be fitted within 48 hours after giving birth.

Male condoms: Men wear this type of contraceptive. Condoms protect both partners from sexually transmitted infections. They are a good choice to have on hand.

Female condoms: Be sure to follow the instructions carefully.

Spermicides: These kill sperm and work best to prevent pregnancy when they are used with a condom. They are known to increase transmission of certain sexually transmitted infections. Follow the directions carefully.

Diaphragms or cervical caps: The opening to the uterus is covered by a diaphragm or cervical cap to prevent sperm from entering. If you used this method of contraception before you became pregnant, you will need to be fitted with a new one, but not until 8 weeks after the birth. Diaphragms work best to prevent pregnancy when they are used along with spermicides.

The following chart shows how most methods of birth control protect against pregnancy:

Contraceptive method	% of women experiencing a pregnancy within the first year of perfect use	% of women experiencing a pregnancy within the first year of typical use
IUC progesterone-releasing (IUS)	0.2	0.2
IUC copper-releasing (IUD)	0.6	0.8
Implant (Implanon)	0.05	0.05
Vasectomy	0.5	0.5
Tubal ligation	0.1	0.15
Progesterone injection (Depo-Provera)	0.2	6
Combined hormonal contraceptive (pill, patch, or ring)	0.3	9
Diaphragm	6	12
Male condom	2	18
Female condom	5	21
Sponge, spermicide	9–20	12–28
Coitus interruptus ("withdrawal")	4	22
Natural family planning (includes LAM)	0.4–5	24
No method	85	

Source: SOGC Contraceptive Guidelines, Revised 2015.

If you have completed your family—sterilization

Sterilization is a permanent birth control operation that can be done on both men and women. Although some sterilizations can be reversed, you and your partner should consider your decision carefully.

The progesterone-releasing IUS provides even higher levels of birth control than tubal ligation, so this is an alternative to a surgical procedure.

Vasectomy: Men can have a simple office procedure known as a *vasectomy*. It is done by a family physician or a urologist (a medical specialist) who cuts the tube (called the *vas deferens*) that carries sperm from the testicles. When this tube is cut, sperm cannot be delivered.

Tubal ligation: There are two ways to block the woman's fallopian tubes so that eggs cannot reach the uterus. One is an operation done in a hospital by a gynaecologist, usually under a general anaesthetic, by using clips or rings, or by burning the tubes. A newer method, done under local anaesthetic, uses small metal coils to block the tubes.

To learn more about birth control, visit www.sexandu.ca.

My personal journal
Your follow-up visit

Your first follow-up visit is usually 6 weeks after the birth. Your baby will likely be checked 2 or 3 days after he is discharged from the birth setting, and may be checked again weekly, or a few times during his first month (see Chapter Eight).

_____

_____

_____

_____

_____

_____

_____

_____

_____

_____

_____

_____

_____

_____

_____

_____

_____

_____

KEEPING TRACK OF MY PROGRESS AFTER BIRTH

Date:

Blood pressure:

Weight:

THINGS TO DISCUSS WITH MY HEALTH CARE PROVIDER

- *The baby blues—signs of postpartum depression*
- *Feelings about my baby*
- *Blood flow*
- *Feelings of pain*
- *Feelings about sex*
- *Birth control (contraception)*
- *Breastfeeding*

Other concerns:

My to-do list:

_____

_____

_____

_____

_____

_____

_____

_____

_____

_____

_____

_____

_____

_____

_____

_____

_____

_____

_____

_____

_____

_____

_____

_____

_____

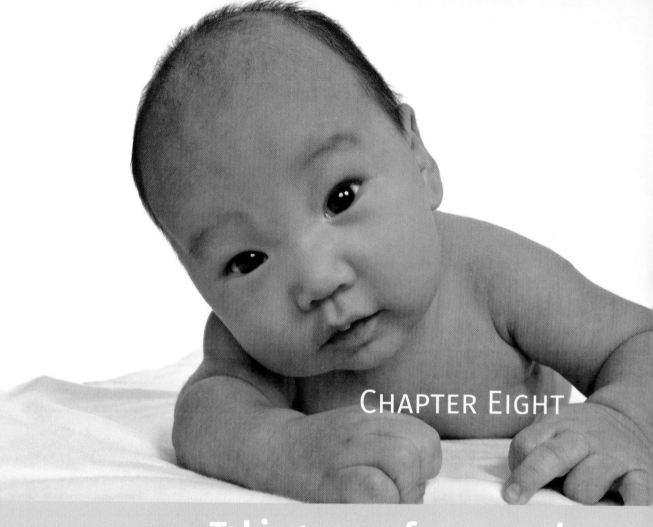

CHAPTER EIGHT

Taking care of your newborn

MAKE SURE YOU REGISTER YOUR BABY'S BIRTH!

Every baby born in Canada must be registered. Ask your health care provider how to do this, or contact Service Canada at 1-800-622-6232 or at www.servicecanada.gc.ca.

Indigenous Canadians may want to look into the Indian Registration and Band Lists program. Information on this program can also be found on the Government of Canada's website at www.aadnc-aandc.gc.ca/eng/1100100021842/1100100021843.

Note: This chapter was reviewed by the Canadian Paediatric Society.

As we begin this second-to-last chapter, congratulations are due—you are now a parent! We hope we have helped answer your questions and prepared you well for the birth of your baby. We trust that you also received the support and help you needed from your support coach and health care team.

We will end this handbook with a few final details about your newborn that will help you start raising a healthy baby. There is lots of information available—just ask your health care provider for suggestions.

So, as we've advised you how to care for your baby in the womb, we have more advice to take you through the first few weeks until you can get more information. For the most part, newborns eat, sleep, and are adored. Oh, and there are diapers, too.

We will begin by telling you about how newborns look. Then, we'll cover some basic first care steps, vaccinations, and the choice of whether to circumcise or not. We'll also focus on diapers, feeding, and sleeping. And, as with all other chapters in this handbook, we'll point out some safety concerns.

First impressions of your baby

Do not be surprised by your baby's appearance at birth and for the first few days. Newborn babies are often covered in a creamy white substance known as *vernix*. When this comes off over time, their skin may be a bit dry and flaky. Many newborns have fine hair called *lanugo* along their backs and shoulders. This usually goes away in a week or two. They may also have white spots, little bruises, marks, rashes, or blotchy skin; all these usually disappear with time.

To fit through the birth canal, a baby's head may have been moulded into an odd shape. Over the next few weeks or months, the baby's head will come back to a more normal shape. You will also feel two soft spots—on the top and at the back of your baby's head (most parents only feel the top spot). These two spots are called **fontanelles** and they are places where the bones of the skull have not grown together yet. These soft spots are normal. Touching them will not harm your baby. The fontanel may pulse up and down a little bit with your baby's heartbeat. This is normal. Vigorous crying may cause the fontanel to bulge slightly; however, it should be flat or slightly depressed when the baby is calm. In most cases, the bones of the skull grow together by the time a baby is 18 months old.

Some newborns have a full head of hair, and others have none. Some babies lose their hair, only to have it grow back a different colour. The colour of your baby's eyes may also change over the next 3 to 6 months.

The hormones in your body at the time of the birth may affect your baby's body. For example, newborns of both sexes may develop swollen breasts when they are a few days old. Some babies' breasts leak a few drops of milk. Do not worry about this milk or try to express it. This is normal, and it will not last. Pregnancy hormones may also make the baby's sex organs larger than normal for a few days. A baby boy may have a reddish scrotum (the sac that holds his testicles), and a baby girl may have a bit of bleeding or white discharge from her vagina. You do not need to be concerned by any of these findings, should they occur.

How to handle your baby safely

Your newborn baby may not be fragile, but you need to handle your baby gently. This keeps him safe and feeling secure.

CARING FOR TWINS AND MULTIPLES

The birth of twins or multiples is an exciting event! You may have already done a lot to prepare yourself for the extra challenge and joys of caring for more than one newborn. Changing diapers, breastfeeding, sleeping, doing laundry . . . all these tasks take on new meaning with twins or multiples. Ask for help. No one expects you to do it all yourself. Set up routines and patterns and then expect them to get broken! Take care of yourself. To learn more about being a parent to twins or multiples, see the Multiple Births Canada website at www.multiplebirthscanada.org.

MUSIC TO THEIR EARS

Talk and sing to your baby throughout your pregnancy, and continue to do so after your baby is born. This fosters bonding between you and your baby and creates a firm foundation for language and literacy skills to build on as your baby grows.

Right from the moment they are born, newborn babies learn how to read signals all around them. They listen to voices, watch faces, and read body language. Babies need to hear and use sounds, sound patterns, and spoken language. This helps prepare them to talk and, eventually, to learn to read printed words.

When you hold your newborn baby, support the head. A baby's neck muscles are weak for the first few months of life. Even though the neck muscles are weak, the muscles in the rest of the body are quite strong! In fact, they are strong enough to allow a squirming baby to move across a surface (where he could fall off), or to wave a fist, or push down his legs to knock a cup of tea or coffee out of your hand.

The best way to prevent any injury or harm is to watch, listen, and stay nearby. When you have to move away from your baby for any reason, put your baby in a safe place, such as the crib. Keep emergency phone numbers close to the phone, just in case. You may wish to take an infant/child first aid and/or CPR (cardio-pulmonary resuscitation) class so you will know what to do in case of an emergency.

Screen-time

The use of smart phones, laptops, televisions, and other electronic devices are part of most people's everyday routine in today's world. Social media can be an effective way for you to share news of your new baby and connect with supports and information. However, they can distract you from your baby. Your baby's first months are a fleeting and important time for both of you. Make sure you spend time away from screens each day to connect with your miraculous newborn. Your baby needs to hear your voice, gaze at your face, and feel safe in your arms in order to feel secure and learn.

Bonding involves two people interacting, sharing, and connecting. So as you respond to your baby's needs, your baby will respond to you. You'll notice that it becomes easier to soothe her, that she wants to be near you, and that she reacts to you even from a distance. Holding, rocking, or talking softly to your baby, all promote bonding.

Safety in your home

- Make sure all the equipment (such as cribs, strollers, and change tables) that you obtain for your newborn meets national safety standards. Go around your house and do a baby safety check.
- Hang crib mobiles high enough so your baby's hands cannot reach them.
- Make sure that bookshelves or other pieces of heavy furniture are securely attached to the wall.
- Install a smoke and carbon monoxide alarm near your baby's room and make sure that all household smoke and carbon monoxide alarms are working. Change the batteries as recommended.
- Never carry a baby and a hot drink at the same time.
- If you need to warm a liquid or food for your baby such as expressed breast milk, always warm it up by putting the container in a pan of hot water. Never use a microwave because the microwave creates hotspots that can burn an infant's mouth.
- Never leave your baby alone with a pet.
- Supervise your baby around brothers and sisters and other young children and around pets.
- Make your home a smoke-free zone. If you do smoke, do it outside and change your clothes afterwards before handling your baby.
- Keep walkways clear of toys and other tripping hazards.
- Ensure emergency contact numbers, including Poison Control, are near the phone or as quick contacts in your cell phone.

Safety around other people

Avoid crowds and crowded places with your newborn when possible. Encourage anyone who wants to hold or play with your baby to wash his or her hands before touching your baby. If people want to kiss the baby, ask them to kiss the top of the head instead of the face.

Encourage close family and those caring for your baby to make sure that their vaccinations, including flu shots, are up-to-date. This creates a cocoon of protection around your newborn until he is old enough to get his own vaccinations.

Safety when you are outdoors

Never leave your baby alone, whether in a car or a stroller or carriage. Do not use sunscreen or insect repellent on your newborn's sensitive skin. Instead, use an insect net and keep your baby in the shade. Use lightweight clothing that keeps skin shaded.

Car seats

Use a rear-facing car seat to travel with your baby in any car. It is safest to use a rear-facing car seat as long as possible. Read the manufacturer's instructions and follow all age, height, and weight specifications.

Keep in mind the following guidelines:

- Only use a car seat with the National Safety Mark label on it. Check the packaging or the back of the car seat for this symbol.
- Follow the directions that come with the car seat for installation and use.
- Install the car seat in the back seat at all times.
- Thread harness straps just at or below your baby's shoulders. The chest clip should be at armpit level, and the harness should fit snugly.

- Look for a car seat clinic where your car seat installation can be double-checked by experts.
- Dress your baby in regular indoor clothing. You can use a blanket on top and a hat for warmth if needed. Snowsuits or bunting bags will interfere with buckling up your baby securely.
- Only use a car seat that is undamaged. Any signs of damage can make a car seat unsafe. It is not safe to use a car seat that has been in a car crash, even a minor one.
- Ensure your baby is never left unattended in a car, even for a short time.
- Be aware of the risk of your baby overheating in a car that is too hot.
- Place car seats on the floor (safest place) and not on the counter, table, or other high places. Car seats are unsteady and can easily fall from high places.
- Use a combination stroller/car seat for public transportation. It is the safest option.

All infant and child car seats sold in Canada must meet Transport Canada's safety regulations. These rules help protect children in case the vehicle stops suddenly or is involved in a crash.

The Government of Canada provides a list of all local places across Canada that inspect and show you how to install and use baby and toddler car sets. Visit www.canada.ca/en/services/transport/road/child-car-seat-safety/child-car-seat-clinics-other-resources.html.

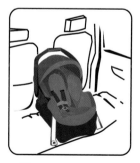

Infant car seat

WHEN TO CALL YOUR HEALTH CARE PROVIDER OR GO TO THE HOSPITAL

Do not wait! Call your health care provider or find a way to go to the hospital safely right away if your baby experiences any of the following:

- *Has a temperature of more than 38.0°C (100.4°F)*
- *Has a seizure (shaking body, arms, and legs)*
- *Has trouble breathing (works hard to suck air in, lips turn a blue-grey colour)*
- *Has pale skin that feels cold and moist*
- *Vomits more than twice in one day (large amounts of vomit, not the usual spit-up)*
- *Has diarrhea (large watery stools) more than twice in one day*
- *Passes blood or blood clots*
- *Wets fewer than four diapers a day after the age of 5 days*
- *Breastfeeds poorly or will not eat*
- *Seems weak, can barely cry*
- *Cries more than usual, cries in a different way, acts very fussy, and nothing you seem to do seems to comfort your baby*

(Continued)

What to expect at your baby's first check-up

Following discharge from the birth setting, a newborn will need to see a health care provider again in 2 to 3 days. If the health care provider is a midwife, she will do a home visit within this time frame. If you have any concerns before this visit, you should contact your health care provider sooner. At this visit, your baby will have a complete physical exam. This includes measuring your baby's weight, height, and head size. Your health care provider will check for signs of jaundice, check how feedings are going, and also talk to you about the basic steps that babies go through as they grow. It's a good idea to bring a list of questions with you.

In many communities, a public health nurse contacts parents after the baby's birth to answer any questions, and in some regions they may set up a time for a home visit. During this visit, the nurse may provide you with information about taking care of both your baby and yourself. Many communities also offer well-baby drop-in clinics where mothers and young babies can come without an appointment—a health care provider can help you find such a clinic.

If you are worried that you or your partner are experiencing postpartum depression, be sure to tell your health care provider, even a paediatrician. Both mothers and fathers can experience depression after the birth of a child.

Some of the symptoms of depression include the following:

- Feeling that you can't care for your baby
- Extreme anxiety or panic attacks
- Trouble making decisions
- Feeling very sad

- Hopelessness
- Feeling out of control*

Getting your baby immunized

Vaccines have been developed to protect babies and children from diseases that can cause serious illness, permanent suffering, or death. Vaccines that are offered to your baby through the public health system are very safe and effective. It's important to make sure your child receives these vaccines at the right times so he can be protected.

The following is a schedule of immunizations that will be offered to your child. The schedule may vary slightly from province to province. The Public Health Agency of Canada provides a list of which immunizations are available in different provinces and territories. See the following website to learn about vaccines in your area of Canada: www.healthycanadians.gc.ca/healthy-living-vie-saine/immunization-immunisation/children-enfants/schedule-calendrier-eng.php.

Keep track of your family's vaccines with Immunize Canada's app: www.immunize.ca/en/app.aspx.

www.caringforkids.cps.ca/handouts/depression_in_pregnant_women_and_mothers

WHEN TO CALL YOUR HEALTH CARE PROVIDER OR GO TO THE HOSPITAL (CONTINUED)

- *Does not act like he or she used to, seems "different" somehow, wakes up less alert, sleeps more than usual*
- *If you are afraid you might hurt your baby*

A healthy baby can get sick very quickly. If you are worried about your baby for any reason, call your health care provider.

Routine immunization schedule for children in Canada						
Age at vaccination	2 months	4 months	6 months	12 months	18 months	4–6 years
Diphtheria Tetanus Pertussis Poliomyelitis	X	X	X		X	X
Hib (Haemophilus influenzae type B)	X	X	X		X	
Rotavirus	2 or 3 doses between 6 weeks and 32 weeks of age					
Mumps Measles Rubella				X	X or X	
Hepatitis B	Infancy or 9–13 years					
Chickenpox (Varicella)				X		X
Pneumococcal	X	X	X	X		
Meningococcal conjugate				X		
Flu	Once a year—all children over 6 months 1-2 doses					

Source: Canadian Paediatric Society, Caring for Kids: www.caring forkids.cps.ca. For a more detailed list, visit www.caringforkids.cps.ca/handouts/vaccination_and_your_child. For information on which vaccines are covered and when in your province, visit: www.healthycanadians.gc.ca/healthy-living-vie-saine/immunization-immunisation/children-enfants/schedule-calendrier-eng.php

Vaccination questions and answers

Are vaccines safe?

Yes. Vaccines are very safe. Serious side effects are rare.

Why do we need vaccines if the diseases they prevent no longer exist?

Most of the diseases we are vaccinated against still exist in Canada and in countries where fewer people are immunized. Outbreaks of the disease do occur. The speed and ease of air travel, with larger numbers of people travelling from or immigrating to Canada, pose a real risk of these diseases being brought into Canada.

Why can't I take a chance that my child will not get sick?

Children who are not vaccinated have a much greater chance of getting the disease than those who have received the vaccine. And they can spread infectious disease to vulnerable persons.

Do vaccines weaken the immune system?

No. Vaccines make the immune system stronger to protect against certain diseases.

Can natural infection be an alternative to vaccines?

Vaccines create immunity to certain diseases without making a person suffer from the disease itself. The diseases children are vaccinated against can cause serious illness with possibility of death or serious disability, so we want to prevent as many people as possible from getting the natural disease.

Jaundice (yellowish skin and eyes)

Jaundice is very common in newborn babies. Baby's skin turns yellow because a high amount of a substance called *bilirubin* is produced

---

VACCINE SAFETY IN CANADA

- *The vaccines used in Canada are very effective and safe.*

- *Serious negative reactions are rare. The dangers of getting the disease itself are many times greater than the risks of serious reactions to the vaccine.*

- *Health authorities around the world are very serious about making sure vaccines are safe.*

- *There is **no** evidence that vaccines cause chronic disease, autism, or sudden infant death syndrome (SIDS). The links that some people say happen—for example, between hepatitis B vaccine and multiple sclerosis— have been proven to be false after scientific study.*

PAIN MANAGEMENT DURING IMMUNIZATION

Immunizations are an important and common health measure in childhood. Parents play a key role in reassuring, soothing and supporting their children. Learn how to reduce your child's stress and pain during immunization at www.immunize.ca/ en/parents/pain.aspx.

or because the liver can't get rid of it quickly enough. You may notice it between 1 and 4 days after your baby is born. Most jaundice is not harmful to your baby and disappears when your baby's body learns to deal with bilirubin. However, a high level of bilirubin, which means severe jaundice, can cause brain damage. It is very important to have your baby checked by your health care provider.

A health care provider can check for jaundice by doing a blood test that measures the bilirubin in your baby's bloodstream. If you had your baby at a hospital, this test may have been done before you left the hospital with your baby.

A health care provider should check your baby on day 2 or 3 for jaundice. This is usually part of the first well-baby visit that you will need to schedule for day 2 or 3 after discharge from your birth setting. In many communities in Canada, a midwife or a nurse does this on an early home visit; however, this service is not available everywhere.

It is uncommon for babies to have such high levels of bilirubin that they are in danger. If you think your baby has jaundice, take the following steps:

- Call your health care provider.
- A baby with jaundice may be sleepier than usual. Feed your baby whenever you see feeding cues and wake your baby if needed to ensure 8 or more feedings in 24 hours. Your baby should be fed both day and night. Dehydration can worsen jaundice. Feeding often will make your baby pass more stool. The milk also gives your baby's liver the energy it needs to process the bilirubin. (For more information on feeding your baby, see page 219.)

Most babies do *not* need hospital treatment for jaundice. However, if the bilirubin test(s) show the need for treatment, it should be done in hospital where the baby will be put under special lights (phototherapy) to reduce jaundice.

If your baby is jaundiced and dehydrated (see "Signs of dehydration in newborns" sidebar on page 211), irritable, has low energy, or has shaking movements that seem like a seizure, go directly to a hospital emergency room.

Circumcision

Circumcision is an operation to remove the skin that covers the head of the penis. An infant must be stable and healthy to be circumcised. It is most often done during the first few days after birth. After a careful review of the medical evidence, the Canadian Paediatric Society does not recommend routine circumcision of every newborn boy. However, parents who decide to circumcise their sons often do so for personal, religious, and cultural reasons. Because circumcision is not essential for health, you should make a decision based on your own values, weighing the benefits and risks. Circumcisions for non-medical reasons are not covered by any provincial and territorial health plans.

It is easy to keep the uncircumcised penis clean by washing the area gently while you are giving your baby boy a bath. The foreskin does not fully pull back (retract) for several years and should never be forced back. Later, when the foreskin fully retracts, your son should be taught to wash gently under it.

Circumcision is an operation that creates some discomfort for the baby. The health care provider performing the circumcision should use some type of local anaesthetic, given by a needle in the area where the circumcision is done. After the circumcision, you can comfort your baby by holding him and breastfeeding him often.

MEDICINES FOR NEWBORNS

Talk to your health care provider before you give your baby any of these:

- *Over-the-counter drugs*

- *Herbal remedies*

- *Vitamins*

Although many are sold without a prescription and are deemed safe, some substances can be harmful, especially to newborns. Always check with your health care provider first.

You will be given instructions on how to look after your baby after the surgery.

Potential benefits of circumcision

A few studies suggest that circumcision may offer the following benefits:

- Less likely to develop cancer of the penis later in life—although this form of cancer is extremely rare
- Less likely to get HIV (human immunodeficiency virus) and HPV (human papillomavirus) infections
- Less likely to get a urinary tract infection during childhood
- Female partners of men who have been circumcised are less likely to get cervical cancer

Potential risks of circumcision

Circumcision is a painful procedure. Problems resulting from the surgery are usually minor. Although serious complications are very rare, they do occur:

- Too much bleeding
- Infection in the area
- Too much skin removed
- Side effects from the method or medicine used for pain relief

The risk of complications is lower in young babies than in older children. To minimize the risks, the procedure should be done by a trained and experienced health care provider using a sterile technique. Someone should follow up with you in the days after the procedure to make sure that bleeding has not increased.

After circumcision, you should contact your health care provider if any of the following occurs:

- Your baby does not urinate within 6 to 12 hours.
- Bleeding lasts for a long time.
- The redness and swelling around the circumcision do not start to go down in 48 hours.

Newborn care

Bowel movements and urine

You can tell if your baby is feeding well by the number of times your baby soils or wets the diaper (see table on page 213). Newborns can get dehydrated very quickly. Dehydration is a drop in the baby's fluid levels. This can cause serious problems. Make sure you are feeding your baby enough (see "When to feed" on page 222) and that your baby has normal amounts of urine and feces, the waste that comes from having a bowel movement (also called *stool*).

Your baby's first bowel movement will look a bit like tar. It will be greenish-black. It's called **meconium.**

- Babies pass meconium for the first day or two after they are born.
- After that, your baby's stool will become looser and greenish-yellow for 3 to 4 days. This is called *transitional stool.*
- Then stools will be yellow, soft, and seedy. Early on, these may come after every feeding. After the first month, stools may not be as frequent (one bowel movement every 2 to 7 days), but they should be soft and yellow.

Check the diaper every time you change your baby to make sure it is wet. If there is plenty of breast milk going in, then plenty of fluid (urine) should be coming out. If your baby's urine is almost clear and hard to see in the diaper (but you can still feel the diaper is

---

SIGNS OF DEHYDRATION IN NEWBORNS

Dehydration (when the body's fluid levels drop) can be very serious.

Call your health care provider or seek medical advice at a local clinic or hospital right away if you see these signs of dehydration:

- *Decreased urination (fewer than four wet diapers in 24 hours in infants or no urine for over 8 hours in older children)*
- *Increased thirst*
- *Absence of tears*
- *Dry skin, mouth, and tongue*
- *Faster heartbeat*
- *Sunken eyes*
- *Greyish skin*
- *Sunken soft spot (fontanelle) on your baby's head*

wet or heavier than a dry diaper), this is a good sign that your baby is getting enough milk. Very yellow urine may mean your baby is dehydrated and needs more milk. If your baby is not feeding well or is showing signs of dehydration seek help. You can:

- Contact your health care provider.
- Contact the breastfeeding centre at your birthing place if they offer that service.
- Search for breastfeeding services near you.

Newborns who lose more than 7% of their total body weight can become very ill. Know the signs of dehydration in newborns (see the sidebar "Signs of dehydration in newborns"). Call your health care provider if you have any concerns or make an appointment to see your baby's doctor if any of the following occurs:

- Your baby wets fewer than four diapers a day after the age of 5 days.
- Your baby isn't feeding well.
- Your baby passes a hard or pellet-like stool or appears to be straining and has trouble passing stool.
- There is blood in your baby's diaper.
- Your baby has diarrhea or starts having many more bowel movements than normal, especially if they are watery and/ or explosive. In newborns, it can be hard to judge whether the stool is actually diarrhea.

Take your baby to the hospital immediately if she has decreased urination (fewer than four wet diapers in 24 hours), especially if she is not feeding well or seems unwell.

Your health care provider will want to know:

- The number of soiled and wet diapers your baby has had
- The amount and colour of the stool you see in the soiled diapers

Baby's age	Average number of wet diapers	Average number of dirty/soiled diapers
Day 1	1/day	1/day
Day 2	2/day	2/day
Day 3	3/day	3/day
Day 4 to 1 month	5 or 6/day	3 or 4/day

After about a month, the number of dirty diapers may change dramatically and almost any amount is normal. Your baby may have several dirty diapers (i.e., stools) a day, or he may go several days without a dirty diaper. The number of dirty diapers will often decrease a bit for breastfed babies after a couple of months. Keep a diary so you know what is normal for your baby and can tell when there has been a significant change.

Source: Canadian Paediatric Society, Caring for Kids: www.caringforkids.cps.ca. April 2013.

Skin care and bathing

Your baby must be kept clean but does not need a full bath every day. Bathing too often can cause your baby's skin to dry out. Bathe your baby every 2 to 3 days or as needed. Your baby can have a full bath even if the cord stump has not fallen off; just pat it dry after the bath. A wet cloth will help keep your baby clean between baths. Wash the face and hands often. Clean the area covered by the diaper after each diaper change. Your newborn baby may have some skin conditions that seem unusual to you. Most are fairly common and do not need to be treated. (See "Common skin rashes" on page 216 for more information.)

You may use mild baby soap to clean the skin. Use an unscented moisturizing cream to soothe dry skin. Pay special attention to the scalp and the folds in your baby's skin.

Bathe your baby in a warm room. Gather all the items you will need first, and take off any jewelry you are wearing that might scratch your baby. Hold your baby securely during the bath.

SAFETY TIPS FOR CHANGING DIAPERS

1. Gather all the items you need before you lay your baby down to be changed:
   - A small washcloth or disposable baby wipes
   - A clean diaper and maybe clean clothes
   - Ointment to prevent diaper rash
2. Never turn your back on your baby, not even for a second!
3. Put your hand on your baby's tummy if you must reach for something. If you cannot reach what you need, take your baby with you.
4. Ignore the doorbell or phone if they happen to ring or take your baby with you to answer them.
5. Avoid using baby powder that can be inhaled by your baby.
6. Wash your hands after each time you change your baby to prevent germs from spreading.
7. Keep the surface where you change your baby's diapers clean.

To keep your baby's skin clean and dry, change your baby each time the diaper is wet or dirty. Most parents find a routine for changing diapers that works for them. For example:

- *Some parents change the baby after each feeding and before they lay the baby down for a nap.*

- *Others find that changing their baby's diaper is a good way to wake up a sleepy baby that still needs to breastfeed from the other breast.*

The best way to prevent diaper rash is to change your baby's diaper often.

Use clean water to wash the eyes, ears, mouth, and face. Do not use cotton swabs to clean inside a baby's nose or ears. You can use a clean washcloth wrapped around your little finger to clean the outer ear and nose. Mucous or earwax will come out by itself in time. Do not use baby oil. It can make your hands and the baby's skin slippery and unsafe.

Start at the top, and work your way down. Wash the face first, then the body, then the bottom. Wipe a girl's genitals from front to back. You do not need to separate the vaginal lips. Keep a baby boy's penis clean by gently washing the area. Do not try to pull back the foreskin—it's usually not safe to do this until a boy is at least 3 to 5 years old.

After you take your baby out of the water, pat your baby completely dry with a towel. Never leave a baby alone in a bathtub, even for 1 second.

Cord care

By 24 to 72 hours after birth, your baby's cord will have started to dry. It should fall off within 1 to 3 weeks. The spot under the stump will become the baby's belly button. Just use plain water to clean your baby's cord stump. Avoid any other liquids.

To keep the cord dry, fold the top of the diaper away from the stump. A small amount of bleeding is normal and you may find a few spots of blood on the undershirt or sleeper. Call your health care provider if your baby has a fever (temperature of 38.0°C [100.4°F] or higher) or if the umbilical area appears red and swollen, oozes yellow pus, or bleeds.

Eye care

Just after your baby was born, your nurse or midwife put medication in each eye to prevent infection from germs that may have entered the eye during the birth. Unless signs of infection appear—such as redness or a discharge from the eye—all you need to do to keep the eyes clean is to wipe each closed eye with a moist cloth. Use a clean corner of a wash cloth for each eye. If you think your baby's eyes are infected, call your health care provider.

Trimming fingernails and toenails

Keeping your baby's nails short will help prevent scratches to your baby's skin. Carefully cut the nails straight across, using fine scissors or baby clippers. You may find it easier to file the nails at first, instead of cutting them. The best time to cut a baby's nails is when she's sleeping.

Dressing

Choose clothing with safety and comfort in mind. Make sure sleepers are snug and there are no drawstrings that could get caught on hooks or knobs.

Outside in the winter, babies may need an undershirt, a shirt, and a sweater, along with warm clothing on their legs, socks or booties, and a snowsuit. Babies lose heat easily, so remember a hat. A good rule of thumb is that your baby will likely need one more layer of clothing than you do to feel comfortable (for example, if you need a shirt and sweater, she may need a shirt, sweater, and jacket). Generally, if her hands and feet are warm, she's warm enough. Check exposed skin frequently.

When using a car seat, dress your baby in regular indoor clothing. You can use a blanket on top and a hat for warmth if needed. Snowsuits or bunting bags will interfere with buckling up your baby securely.

In the summer, babies may be most comfortable in only a T-shirt and diaper. A clue that your baby may be too warm is if the back of

HOW TO PREVENT DIAPER RASH

The best way to prevent diaper rash is to change your baby's diaper often, especially if your baby has diarrhea. If your child has diarrhea, you can also help to prevent diaper rash with an unscented barrier cream to protect the skin.

HOW TO TREAT DIAPER RASH

- *When you change your baby's diaper, wash her bottom with mild soap and warm water (just water if there is no stool), rinse, and pat dry. If the skin is really sore and red, it may be less painful to wash the area in a warm bath.*

- *Use an unscented barrier ointment, such as petroleum jelly or a cream with zinc oxide, to protect and lubricate the area after each diaper change. If you use a cream, clean it off with soap and water after each change and reapply. Do not share creams and ointments*

(Continued)

her neck is hot, damp, or clammy. In air-conditioned rooms or cars, your baby may need more clothes than you do, because he is less active. Babies tend to feel cold sooner than you would.

Common skin rashes

Your newborn baby may have some skin rashes or spots that do not seem to be normal to you. Most are very common and do not need to be treated.

Baby acne is a red, pimply rash on the face. It usually goes away over time.

Milia are tiny whiteheads on your baby's face. They will also go away over time.

Erythema toxicum is a common splotchy red rash that tends to come and go on different parts of a newborn's body. It is most common on the second or third day of life, but it can appear at birth or within the first 2 weeks. Each splotch might have firm yellow or white bumps surrounded by a flare of red. They may stay for only a few hours or for several days. They will slowly disappear.

Cradle cap looks like greasy scales on the baby's scalp. There might be some redness around the scales and on other parts of the baby's body—such as in the folds of the neck, armpits, behind the ears, on the face, and in the diaper area. This usually goes away on its own.

Diaper rash is a red rash in the diaper area. It is caused when urine or stool in the diaper makes the baby's skin tender and red. You can help prevent diaper rash by changing your baby's diaper often. (See the "How to prevent diaper rash" and "How to treat diaper rash" sidebars.)

Candida diaper rash appears around the genitals and buttocks and is very red with small red spots close to the red patches. It is a type of yeast infection that can also appear in the baby's mouth. When it's in the mouth, it's called **thrush.** If you think your baby has a candida infection, see your health care provider. Candida rashes need to be treated with a prescription cream.

Heat rash usually happens during hot and humid weather or in winter if your baby wears too many layers of clothing. It causes little red bumps on the skin—mostly in the folds of a baby's skin or on parts of the body where clothing fits snugly. You can help prevent or treat heat rash by taking off extra clothing and by keeping your baby cool by dressing him in loose-fitting, light cotton clothing (especially in warm, humid weather).

Contact dermatitis is a rash that occurs when your baby's skin comes into contact with something that irritates the skin or something that he is allergic to (such as snaps on clothing or dyes in clothing). In most cases, it only appears on the part of the skin that came in contact with the item your baby is allergic to. Tell your health care provider if this happens. You may be asked if your baby has come into contact with anything new to find the cause of the rash.

Eczema is a skin rash that shows up as dry, thick, scaly skin or tiny red bumps that can blister, ooze, or become infected if they are scratched. It appears most often on a baby's forehead, cheeks, or scalp, but it can also occur on other parts of the body. It may happen in babies who have allergies or a family history of allergy or eczema. There is no cure for eczema, but it can be controlled and often will go away after several months or years. Talk to your health care provider if you think your baby has eczema.

Ways to prevent a flat head

Babies who always sleep on their back with their head to the same side can develop flat spots. This is not dangerous and will not

---

HOW TO TREAT DIAPER RASH (CONTINUED)

with other children and don't touch the affected skin and then put your fingers back into the jar. Use a different finger if you need more ointment.

- Using wipes can dry out your baby's skin. If you use wipes, be sure they are alcohol-free and unscented.

- Do not use baby powder or talc.

- If possible, keep your baby's diaper off for short periods to expose her skin to open air. This can help your baby feel better and heal the rash faster.

Source: Canadian Paediatric Society, Caring for Kids: www.caringforkids.cps.ca. September 2013.

affect a baby's brain or development. In most cases, it goes away on its own. You can also prevent your baby from getting a flat spot by changing the placement of your baby's head each day:

- Place your baby with the head at the top of the crib one day so that she must turn in one direction to look out into the room.
- The next day, place her head at the foot of the crib so that she must turn her head in the other direction to look out into the room. Change your baby's direction in the crib each day.
- Have "tummy time" when your baby is awake, several times a day starting as soon as the baby is born. You don't need to wait until the cord falls off. You must supervise your baby at all times! Lay your baby on her tummy while you are present and talk or sing to her.

Sleeping in a safe environment[*]

Your baby needs lots of sleep to stay healthy, happy, and growing, so where your baby sleeps is important. If you create a safe place for your baby to sleep, you will reduce the risk of injuries and the risk of **sudden infant death syndrome (SIDS)**. SIDS is when a baby under 12 months old dies unexpectedly while sleeping. No one knows what causes SIDS, but studies show that there are some simple things that you can do to help reduce the chances of SIDS (see "Ways to reduce the risk of SIDS" sidebar).

For the first 6 months, the safest way for your baby to sleep is on her back in a crib in your room. This is called ***room sharing*** and may help protect against SIDS. Since 2016, Health Canada has banned the sale of drop-side cribs because of injury potential. Babies should never be placed to sleep on standard beds, water beds, air

[*] *Canadian Paediatric Society, www.caringforkids.cps.ca/handouts/safe_sleep_for_babies, July 2016.*

mattresses, couches, futons, or armchairs. It is not safe for a baby to sleep for a long period in a seated or semi-reclined position. If your baby falls asleep in the car seat, swing, stroller, or so on, supervise him closely and move him to a crib, cradle, or bassinet as soon as possible.

No bedmates

Keep your baby in a crib in your room until your baby is at least 6 months old. This is an excellent set-up because you are close and can breastfeed easily without actually sharing a bed. Adult beds are not designed for infants. They can be unsafe.

• A baby can get trapped between the mattress and the wall or the bed frame.
• A baby can fall off the bed.
• An adult or older child can roll over and suffocate a baby.
• Soft bedding can cover the baby's head and cause overheating or suffocation.

If you are considering bed sharing with your baby, talk with your health care provider or public health nurse to learn how to reduce the risks.

Feeding your baby

The time you spend feeding your baby is a special time for both of you. Babies thrive on being held close. Many new mothers feel a close bond forming with their babies when they feed them.

Breast milk is the best and only food for babies for the first 6 months. The Society of Obstetricians and Gynaecologists of Canada, the Canadian Paediatric Society (CPS), Dietitians of Canada (DC), Health Canada, the United Nations Children's Fund (UNICEF), and the World Health Organization (WHO) all recommend this as the best way to feed babies. After 6 months of only breastfeeding, when baby is showing signs of readiness, parents can begin to give

BREASTFEEDING IS THE MOST HEALTHY AND NATURAL WAY TO FEED YOUR BABY

REMEMBER:

The colostrum made by your breasts in the first few days after birth is the perfect food for your new baby. Although your breasts produce only a small amount of colostrum, it is enough. You do not need to give your baby anything else.

A daily vitamin D supplement of 400 IU is recommended by Health Canada for all exclusively and partially breastfed infants, from birth to 2 years of age.

Talk to your health care provider or community health nurse about your child's vitamin D needs and how to meet them.

the child other foods, while still breastfeeding (until your child is 2 years old or even older). Breast milk contains antibodies, growth factors, enzymes, and other things that affect your baby's short- and long-term health. No type of formula has these benefits.

The decision to feed infant formula should be made carefully. Formula differs from breast milk but provides the basic nutrition for baby to grow. If you want to breastfeed and are feeding infant formula, be sure to talk with your health care provider, who will help you or refer you to someone who can help you with breastfeeding.

If there is a medical reason to feed infant formula or you have made an informed decision to formula feed your baby, it is important to know how to select, prepare, feed, and store infant formula. Formula must be prepared correctly, feeding equipment must be sanitized properly, and once opened, a can of formula must be stored safely. Formula can be recalled because of safety concerns and recall information can be found on the Health Canada's website at www.hc-sc.gc.ca/ahc-asc/media/advisories-avis/index-eng.php.

It is also very important that you learn your baby's hunger cues, how to feed your baby at his pace so he is comfortable while feeding, and to know the signs when he is full and the feeding should end. Always hold your baby during feedings and make feeding a pleasant time for the both of you. Talk to your health care provider to learn more about formula feeding.

Breastfeeding

Breast milk includes the special milk called colostrum, the first milk produced. It has all the right ingredients in just the right amounts to help your baby grow. It is the perfect temperature, and it is always available. Breastfeeding helps you feel close to your baby, and it is important for your baby to feel close to you.

Colostrum made in your breasts is a yellowish sticky milk-like substance rich in vitamins, protein, and antibodies to protect your baby from infections. Newborns have fat and water stored in their bodies. They use this up in the first day of life. This explains why newborns lose weight at first. Colostrum alone is enough food for your baby for the first few days. There is no need to give your baby water or formula. The amount of milk you produce will increase within 2 to 3 days.

All mothers should eat well and follow the Canada Food Guide for their own health and well-being. Breastfeeding women need more calories. Include an extra two to three Food Guide servings each day. Eating well helps you recover from the baby's birth and helps your body heal. It will also give you extra calories for energy to look after your baby. However, even if you are not eating a healthy diet, breastfeeding is still the best way to feed your baby.

When to start

The best time to start breastfeeding is immediately after the baby is born, within the first hour, when the baby is placed against the mother's skin in what is called *skin-to-skin contact*. Skin-to-skin should be done for at least the first hour or until the baby has been breastfed and as long as the mother wishes. Your nurse or midwife will help you to get started. Skin-to-skin contact helps both you and your baby with two important things: bonding and breastfeeding. Baby, when placed skin-to-skin on mother's semi-reclined body, will instinctively find the mother's breast.

Not all babies know how to breastfeed right away. It is still a good idea to use this time to get breastfeeding started. Make sure you let the hospital staff members know that you want your baby to stay in your room with you (rooming in) so you can breastfeed your baby whenever he seems hungry. When together, mother and baby can get to know one another and mother can learn to recognize and respond to her baby's cues. Feeding your baby often helps to increase your milk supply.

When to feed

Feed your baby whenever she shows hunger cues. It is always best to respond to early cues such as baby stirring, turning head and rooting, putting hands to mouth, licking lips, and making sucking movements. Waiting until your baby shows late signs of hunger, such as crying, can make feeding more difficult. Babies should feed 8 or more times in 24 hours. Some feedings may last longer than others. Your baby needs to feed at night as well as during the daytime. Keeping baby with you will help you see her feeding cues and you can respond right away. This will help both of you enjoy feeding time.

Breastfeeding positions

You can breastfeed your baby in many comfortable positions. Here are a few suggestions.

Laid-back breastfeeding

Find a bed or couch where you can lean back and be well supported—not flat, but comfortably leaning back so that when you put your baby on your chest, gravity will keep him in position with his body moulded to yours. Have your head and shoulders well supported. Let your baby's whole front touch your whole front. Because you're leaning back, you don't have a lap, so your baby can rest on you in any position you like. Just make sure her whole front is against you.

Lying down

Lie in bed on your side, with your head on a couple of pillows. Lay your baby down beside your lower breast.

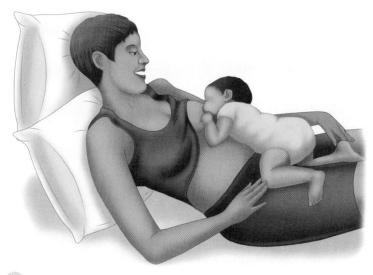

Laid-back breastfeeding

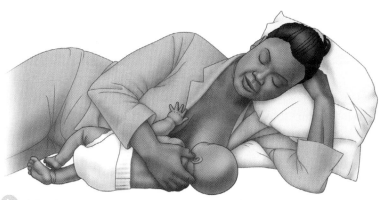

Lying down

Adapted and reproduced with permission of Public Health, Region of Peel.

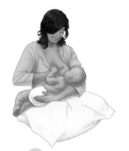

Cradle hold

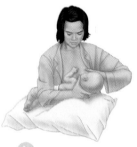

Cross cradle hold

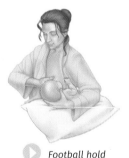

Football hold

Adapted and reproduced with permission of Public Health, Region of Peel.

Cradle hold

Find a comfortable sitting position. Prop a pillow under the arm that holds your baby. Put your baby's head at your breast with your baby's feet lying across your abdomen.

Cross cradle hold

Find a comfortable sitting position. Prop a pillow under the arm that holds your baby. Support your baby at the base of his head and neck using the arm opposite to the breast that will be used. Support your baby's back and buttocks with your forearm. Your baby's ear, shoulder, and hip should be in a straight line with his stomach touching your stomach.

Football hold

Find a comfortable sitting position. Tuck your baby's legs under your arm so the feet point toward your back. Use a pillow to support your baby's head at the level of your breast. (This position puts less pressure on your abdomen if you had a caesarean birth.)

How to get started

Step 1: Get comfortable

Use pillows to support your arm. Hold your baby close and point the face toward your breast. Bring your baby toward you. Do not go toward your baby. If you do, you may have back pain and an uncomfortable latch.

Step 2: Latching on

Getting a comfortable latch or attachment to the breast is one of the most important parts of breastfeeding. Here are some tips to help you:

- Roll your baby's body toward you and wait until her mouth opens.
- Point your nipple toward your baby's nose. When bringing your baby toward your breast, support her neck and shoulders. Do not push on her head. Once your baby is latched, the chin—not the nose—will touch your breast.
- Put your baby onto the breast with the lower jaw well down on the areola (the dark area around the nipple) and lots of your nipple in the mouth.
- This way, your baby will not be sucking from the nipple but applying pressure with the jaws and tongue further back. This will allow milk to flow from the milk ducts around the nipple into her mouth.

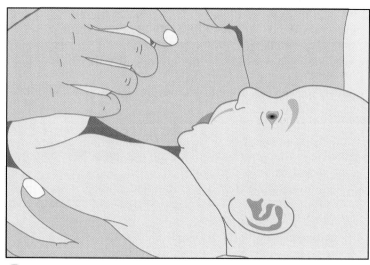

A comfortable and correct latch

Step 3: Breaking the suction

To take your baby off your breast, slide your smallest finger inside the corner of the mouth and push down gently to break the suction seal. Then go back to Step 2 and try to get your baby to latch on again.

Breastfeeding tips

- Make sure your baby is latching on in the correct way and that you feel comfortable during breastfeeding. Ask for help if needed.
- Be sure to drink water whenever you feel thirsty.
- Get into a comfortable position before you begin breastfeeding.
- Being skin-to-skin with your baby in the early days will help the breastfeeding process.
- Keep your baby close to you so you can see and hear his feeding cues (stirring, mouth opening, rooting, and hands or fingers to mouth) as soon as possible.
- Start with one breast, letting your baby breastfeed for as long as he likes.
- Your baby will fall asleep, stop sucking, or let go of your breast when finished.
- If your baby falls asleep too quickly on your breast, try using breast compression to help him to drink more.
- Make sure that your baby is not too hot (wearing too many clothes) while breastfeeding.
- Take a break. Burp your baby if needed. Change a soiled diaper and wash your hands. (This often helps the baby to wake up and continue feeding.)
- Start again with the other breast. If he won't take any more, try to remember to start with this breast next time.
- Try starting with a different breast at each feeding.

- Offer both breasts at every feeding. Sometimes your baby may decide to feed from only one breast at a feeding. The more milk that flows from the breast at each feeding, the more milk you will make.
- Feed your baby often at first to help the amount of milk increase and to prevent your breasts from being engorged.
- Some babies have growth spurts around 3, 6, and 12 weeks. They will ask to be fed more often for 24 to 48 hours. This is nature's way of helping you to produce more milk.
- Taking care of a newborn is tiring. If possible, ask for help with your errands, housework, and other children.

Expressing breast milk

Learn how to express your breast milk by gently massaging or pushing on your breast with your hand or with a breast pump. You can do this when you want to rub a few drops of milk on your nipple, to soften your areola, or to store milk to let someone else feed the baby when you cannot be with her. How to express milk with your hands:

- Wash your hands, get comfortable, and have a clean or sterile container ready to collect the milk.
- Massage your breasts with both hands.
- Place your thumb and first finger on the edge of the areola while supporting your breast with the rest of your hand.
- Push gently back toward your chest wall.
- Roll your fingers and thumb toward the nipple while you also apply slight pressure.
- Release the pressure and repeat this step in a rhythmic motion.
- Continue until the flow of milk has slowed down or stopped.
- Rotate your hand to remove milk from all areas of the breast then repeat all steps with the second breast.

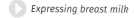

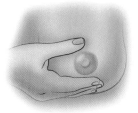

Expressing breast milk

Press (back towards your chest)

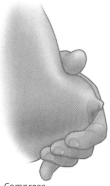

Compress

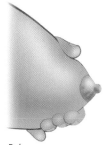

Relax

227

Don't worry if you only get a few drops of milk at first. This skill becomes easier and more efficient with practice. You can also express your milk using a manual or electric breast pump.

Seal the container that contains your breast milk. Put a label on it with the date and time. Do not add warm milk to already cooled or frozen milk. Cool the newly expressed milk first, before adding it to older stored milk.

You can store breast milk safely in these ways:

Freshly expressed breast milk at room temperature (16–29°C)	*3–4 hours*
Fresh milk in refrigerator (≤ 4°C)	*72 hours*
Cooler with a freezer pack	*24 hours*
Deep freezer (≤ -17°C)	*6–12 months*
Throw out all milk that is older than the above storage times!	

Source: Academy of Breastfeeding Medicine. Clinical Protocol Number #8: Human Milk Storage Information for Home Use for Full Term Infants. (Original Protocol March 2004; Revision #1 March 2010.)

Common breastfeeding problems

Tender, sore breasts

The best way to care for your breasts is to make sure that your baby latches deeply and that you are comfortable at every feeding. Change breastfeeding positions to remove milk from all parts of your breasts. Make sure both breasts get a balanced amount of breastfeeding time. Wearing a full-support breastfeeding bra that fits you well, even at night, may help.

Sore nipples

During the first couple of weeks of breastfeeding, it is common for your nipples to feel tender when your baby first latches on to the breast. You should feel more comfortable once you and your baby learn to work together to get a deep latch. It is important to have someone skilled with helping breastfeeding mothers work with you if breastfeeding is painful.

The most common cause of sore nipples is incorrect positioning and a shallow latch. If you notice a tender feeling when your baby latches, count to 10 and see if the discomfort lessens. If it doesn't, then use your finger and gently enter your baby's mouth to break the seal. Reposition your baby and try to latch again. Both you and your baby should be comfortable when breastfeeding. If you have nipple pain throughout the feeding or after the feeding, this is a sign that something is wrong. Seek help right away. Check with the hospital nurse or the public health nurse for more information.

Breast milk has healing properties and applying a few drops to your nipples before and after breastfeeding can provide comfort. If you use breast pads to absorb leaking milk, make sure you change them whenever they become damp. Avoid using soap on your nipples. Soap will wash away your natural breast lubricants.

Engorgement

Breasts become engorged (hard, lumpy, and painful) when they become overly full. You can prevent engorgement by breastfeeding often. Watch your baby for early feeding cues and be sure to breastfeed eight or more times in 24 hours. Be sure to breastfeed during the night as well as during the daytime.

If your breasts become engorged try placing a cold compress on each breast between feedings, and just before breastfeeding apply a warm compress to help the milk begin to flow. Gently massaging the breast, moving your hand from the chest wall toward the nipple, can also help the milk to flow. If your nipple looks flat and the skin feels tight, you can hand express some milk to soften the area and make it easier for your baby to latch. Another way that you can make the areola softer around the base of the nipple is reverse pressure softening. One way to do this is by using your fingers to apply gentle pressure around the base of the nipple, pushing inward toward the chest. Repeat the motion moving your fingers around the areola until you feel the tissue become softer.

If you are unable to get your baby to latch and your breasts continue to feel engorged, be sure to call someone skilled with helping breastfeeding mothers. Unrelieved engorgement can be painful and lead to other breastfeeding concerns.

Blocked milk ducts

If you notice a tender area of the breast with possible redness, swelling, and warmth, you may have a blocked milk duct. Sometimes a lump can be felt if the blockage is close to the skin surface. Blocked milk ducts are more common when breastfeeding is infrequent and too much milk is in the breast. Pressure on that part of the breast by a tight bra, the strap of a baby carrier, and so on can also trigger a blocked milk duct.

Applying warm compresses before the feeding and gently massaging the breast, moving your hands toward the nipple, can help move the blockage. Position your baby so that baby's chin points in the direction of the firm area if possible. Breastfeeding will usually help the blockage clear. If your blocked duct persists or if feedings are uncomfortable and you are unsure if your baby is latching deeply, be sure to have someone skilled with helping breastfeeding mothers observe you feeding your baby. They can likely provide you with some helpful tips.

Mastitis

Mastitis is an inflammation of the breast and can be accompanied by an infection. Mothers with mastitis are usually fatigued, feel a tender area in the breast, and have a flu-like muscular aching. Later, a fever and chills can develop and the tender area of the breast can become red and warm. Mastitis is more likely to happen when the breast becomes too full and breastfeeding is infrequent. Skin breakdown from sore nipples can also lead to the development of mastitis, so it is always important to get help right away if breastfeeding is feeling uncomfortable.

If you think that you have mastitis, keep breastfeeding because frequent and thorough milk removal is necessary. The milk will not harm your baby. If it is too painful to breastfeed, then try to remove milk from your breast using hand expression or a breast pump. Gently massaging the breast while your baby is breastfeeding or when you are hand expressing or pumping can also help the milk to flow. Rest whenever you can. Analgesics such as acetaminophen and ibuprofen can be taken and are not harmful to your baby. Contact your health care provider if you think that you have mastitis. You may require an antibiotic to treat the infection.

What if I cannot breastfeed?

The vast majority of mothers can breastfeed. For some mothers, breastfeeding is not an option. Feeding expressed milk or milk from a human milk bank may be an option. Talk to your health care provider for more information.

If breastfeeding or feeding breast milk are not options, using a store-bought, cow milk-based, iron-fortified infant formula for the first 9 to 12 months can provide the necessary calories and nutrients.

To learn more about choosing formula and the safe preparation, feeding, and storage of formula, talk to your health care provider or contact your local public health office.

Cleaning pumps and infant feeding supplies

Feeding supplies and breast pump parts must be clean before each use. They should be sterilized in boiling water for 2 minutes and then air-dried before use or storage. All infant feeding equipment should be covered until ready for use.

For more information, visit Health Canada's website at www.hc-sc .gc.ca/fn-an/nutrition/infant-nourisson/pif-ppn-recommandations-eng.php.

Spitting up (reflux)

Spitting up or gastroesophageal reflux (GER) or regurgitation is one of the most common infant conditions. All babies spit up to some extent. Spitting up happens because the ring of muscle surrounding an infant's esophagus as it enters the stomach is still immature in the first months of life. When infants burp up swallowed air, milk escapes at the same time because this muscle is weak; this is called *reflux*. Spitting up may go on for hours after a feeding. It usually decreases as an infant gets older and this muscle ring gets stronger. Spitting up tends to peak at 4 months, and most infants stop spitting up by about 12 months of age.

Spitting up is rarely an indication that a baby has an allergy or intolerance to any food or milk. Only rarely will an infant bring up enough milk to reduce caloric intake and slow normal weight gain. Parents will need to discuss severe spitting up with their health care provider if it persists past a child's first birthday, if their child resists normal feedings, or if the reflux is green in colour. These symptoms may be from other and less common conditions such as gastroesophageal reflux disease, or GERD.

If your doctor diagnoses your baby with GERD, she may recommend keeping your baby upright for 20 to 30 minutes after feeding and elevating the head of the bed by 30 degrees. Never elevate the mattress by modifying it in any way with pillows or wedges, because this can create an entrapment risk. Instead, elevate the end of the crib by placing blocks or books on the floor under the crib legs.

Why babies cry

Crying and "colic"

Healthy babies cry. It is the way they express their needs and communicate with the people around them. Most of the time, parents respond with what their baby needs by offering food, helping their baby sleep, changing a diaper, skin-to-skin, or just cuddling. If you look at it that way, crying is quite useful for babies who depend on other people to meet all of their needs.

There are times when even the most caring parent cannot soothe a baby's cries. Know that it's not your fault.

When a baby cries long and hard (without a break) even though he has been fed, changed, and cuddled, the baby is said to be "colicky." For a long time, people thought that colic was a health problem that some babies had and others did not.

New information suggests that what used to be called colic is really a normal part of being a baby. All babies go through a time early in life when they cry more than at any other time. This is sometimes called "the period of purple crying."

Each baby is different. During this time of heavy crying—which happens most often between 3 and 8 weeks—some babies may cry much more than others. Their crying may seem stronger, and it may be harder (sometimes impossible!) to soothe.

NEVER, NEVER SHAKE YOUR BABY!

Shaking can damage your baby's brain. It may even kill him. No child should ever be shaken.

WALK AWAY.

CALL FOR HELP.

This is normal and there is no lasting effect on your baby. It will not last forever. This time of intense (and unexplained) crying can end as quickly as it started, or it may slowly decrease over time. In most cases, it ends by the time your baby is 3 to 4 months old.

In the meantime, there are some tips to help you get through a stressful time. (Refer to the section "What can parents do to help soothe a crying baby?")

Why do some babies cry more than others?

Some experts believe that babies who cry more than others are more sensitive by nature and have a hard time controlling their crying. They may have more trouble soothing themselves and getting settled into their natural body rhythms when they are very young.

In general, studies show that there is nothing wrong with the bowels of babies who cry long and hard. Nor is there strong evidence that the crying is caused by gas, wind, or food allergies. In fact, crying causes infants to swallow air, which they burp up or pass as wind. Because they strain and tighten their stomach muscles, this also forces air out of the rectum.

What can parents do to help soothe a crying baby?

Each baby is unique, and what helps soothe one baby may not work for others. The hard part for parents is to find what works for their baby. Be aware that there may be times when nothing works.

Here are some ideas to help calm your baby or prevent crying at times when he is fussy:

- Check to see if the crying is a sign that your baby needs something—a diaper change, a feeding, relief from being too hot or too cold, or needing more or less stimulation.

- Holding skin-to-skin, hugging, and cuddling will not spoil your baby. Hold your baby. Turn off the lights and keep the room quiet. Too much noise or action can often trigger crying or make it worse.
- Soft music, white noise, or a gentle shushing noise can soothe some babies.
- Many babies are soothed by motion. Try walking with your baby in a quality carrier or in a stroller. Rock or sway your baby in a gentle, rhythmic motion. Or try going for a ride in the car.
- Sucking sometimes helps babies to calm down and relax. Offer to breastfeed your baby.
- Give your baby a warm bath.
- Do not tie anything around your baby's neck or fasten anything to your baby's clothing with a cord that could get caught around your baby's neck. This could cause choking or strangulation.

Only do gentle and soothing things to comfort your baby. Never shake your baby. If you are feeling upset by the crying or feel frustrated that your efforts are not helping, put the baby in a safe place (such as her crib) and take a moment to calm yourself.

Call your doctor if:

- Your baby is not behaving as usual and is not eating or sleeping.
- Your baby has a fever.
- Your baby is vomiting, has diarrhea, or has blood in his stool.
- Your baby could be hurt from a fall or injury.
- Your baby cries excessively after 3 months of age.
- You are afraid you might hurt your baby.

Where can you go for help?

The early days of taking care of a new baby can be difficult. You may not be sleeping much and you will be focusing on meeting your baby's needs 24 hours a day.

HOW TO SWADDLE A BABY

Some people like to swaddle to help calm a baby. Swaddling is controversial because of the risk of missing feeding cues or overheating, and tight swaddling can lead to hip dysplasia. If you choose to swaddle your baby, it is safer if you follow these directions:

1. *Follow your infant's cues and don't wrap if your infant resists.*

2. *Use a lightweight blanket and dress your infant in a light sleeper or onesie to avoid overheating.*

3. *When you swaddle your infant ensure he can flex his legs and that his head is uncovered. Your infant should be swaddled in a way that his hands are free from the blanket. He should be able to show feeding cues such as sucking on his hands.*

4. *Stop swaddling when your baby shows signs of rolling over.*

Talk to your health care provider about swaddling your infant.

See page 218 for information on sleeping in a safe environment.

A baby's constant crying can be stressful. The most important thing to know is that it is not your fault. And it will get better. In the meantime, be sure to take care of yourself.

Arrange for child care relief so you can get some rest. Find a friend, family member, or someone else you trust who can look after your baby for short periods while you get a break. If people offer to help, accept.

- It sounds simple, but eating and sleeping well can make a big difference in how well you can cope. Try to get at least 3 hours of sleep in a row, twice a day.
- Sometimes you may have negative thoughts. That's okay as long as you do not act on those thoughts. If you feel depressed, angry, anxious, or worried, or if the negative thoughts persist, talk to someone you trust and get help.
- Many community resources offer support to parents, especially new mothers. If you are not sure where to go, talk to your paediatrician, family doctor, or public health nurse.

What about soothers (pacifiers)?

When your baby is showing signs that he wants to suck, it could mean that your baby is hungry, even if a feeding was only a short time ago. Offer a breast and see if your baby is interested in feeding. The stimulation of baby sucking can help your body make more milk, and this is especially helpful during growth spurts.

If your baby is fussy, there are many ways to soothe your baby without offering a soother. Try holding your baby skin-to-skin or cuddling. Rocking your baby, singing, and even taking your baby for a car ride can help sometimes.

If you are considering giving your baby a soother, be sure to talk to your health care provider about the risks. Soothers can interfere with the success of breastfeeding. Research also has shown that soothers are associated with a higher risk of ear infections and prolonged use can lead to dental problems. There are also safety precautions that you need to know if you decide to give your baby a pacifier.

- Limit the time your baby uses a soother.
- Make sure the pacifier is clean and not damaged.
- Never dip the pacifier in sugar or honey.
- Never tie a pacifier around your baby's neck.[*]

Parenting classes

Classes to promote good parenting skills are offered in most communities. These classes are good for every new parent because they help boost your knowledge and confidence. The best thing they offer new parents is a chance to share their experience with other parents who have many of the same problems and joys. The classes are very useful and helpful for first-time parents.

In these classes, you will learn basic parenting skills, such as feeding, how to change a diaper, and bathing. You'll also talk about other topics, such as child safety, sibling rivalry, and coping with frustration. If you and your partner came to Canada recently from another country, parenting classes may help you learn more about raising a child in Canada.

First aid and infant CPR (cardio-pulmonary resuscitation) courses are also available. To learn more about these courses and how

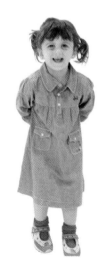

*Adapted from the Canadian Paediatric Society, "Pacifiers (soothers): A User's Guide for Parents." For more information on soothers and other tips about caring for your baby, go to the Canadian Paediatric Society's website for parents at www.caringforkids.cps.ca.

to register, contact the Canadian Red Cross, Heart and Stroke Foundation, or your public health unit.

Here we are, at the end of our role—getting you through your pregnancy and off to a positive start. So, please accept our best wishes for a long healthy life for you and the newest member of your family. Happy baby!

CHAPTER NINE

Finding help

Key resources and services

Most people have questions about pregnancy and the growth of their baby. This section provides key resources and services about your health, before and during pregnancy and in the first few weeks after your baby is born. The list includes helpful websites, documents, programs, and phone numbers that will help you find answers to your questions or learn more about having a healthy pregnancy and baby.

Abuse (violence)

Assaulted Women's Helpline
Crisis line with help in 150 languages that is open 24 hours a day, 7 days a week.
1-866-863-0511

Shelters
To find a safe place to stay, for counselling, or to have information to develop a safety plan for you and your children.
www.sheltersafe.ca

Alcohol and drug use

All provinces and territories have programs for people with alcohol and other drug problems. Ask your health care provider.

Alcohol and Pregnancy
The Public Health Agency of Canada's website provides information about alcohol and pregnancy.
www.phac-aspc.gc.ca/hp-gs/guide/03_ap-ag-eng.php

Alcohol-Free Pregnancy
The Best Start Resource Centre's website provides information about alcohol and pregnancy.
www.alcoholfreepregnancy.ca

Canadian Centre on Substance Abuse
Changes lives by bringing people and knowledge together to reduce the harm of alcohol and other drugs on society.
1-613-235-4048 or www.ccsa.ca

Drug and Alcohol Helpline
Free health services information.
1-800-565-8603 or www.drugandalcoholhelpline.ca

Motherisk
Information and guidance for pregnant or breastfeeding women about risks associated with drug, chemical, infection, disease, and radiation exposures. Information on alcohol and substance use in pregnancy.
1-877-327-4636 or www.motherisk.org

Bereavement (grief)

Baby's Breath
Prevents sudden and unexpected infant deaths and stillbirths by advocating for and supporting research, disseminating information, and providing bereavement support to families.
1-800-363-7437 or www.babysbreathcanada.ca

Pregnancy and Infant Loss Network
Offers support and hope in dealing with pregnancy and infant loss.
1-888-301-7276 or www.pailnetwork.ca

Breastfeeding

Breastfeeding Committee for Canada
Protects, promotes, and supports breastfeeding in Canada as the normal method of infant feeding.
www.breastfeedingcanada.ca

Breastfeeding Information for Parents
An interactive breastfeeding course for parents.
www.breastfeedinginfoforparents.ca

Breastfeeding Information When You Need It (WYNI): App

Windsor-Essex County Health Unit breastfeeding app for Android and iPhone devices.
www.wechu.org/feeding-your-baby/wyni-breastfeeding-information-when-you-need-it

Canadian Human Rights Commission

Provide equal opportunity to everyone in Canada and to help people confront discrimination in their daily lives.
1-888-214-1090 or www.chrc-ccdp.ca

International Breastfeeding Centre

Information and short video clips about breastfeeding.
www.ibconline.ca

La Leche League Canada

Information and support for breastfeeding.
1-800-665-4324 or www.lllc.ca

Ontario Breastfeeding Services (Bilingual, Online)

Search for breastfeeding services near you.
www.ontariobreastfeeds.ca

Child health and development

AboutKidsHealth

The Hospital for Sick Children—AboutKidsHealth website goal is to improve the health and well-being of children in Canada and world-wide by making paediatric health care information available around the globe and in multiple languages.
www.aboutkidshealth.ca

Best Start Resource Centre

Online resources about preconception health, prenatal health, and early child development.
www.beststart.org

Canadian Association of Family Resource Programs

Parenting resources, including a directory of family resource programs across Canada.
1-866-637-7226 or www.frp.ca and www.parentsmatter.ca

Canadian Partnership for Children's Health and Environment

Resources with information on how to protect children's health from environmental pollutants and toxic chemicals.
www.healthyenvironmentforkids.ca

Caring for Kids

Child and teen health information from the Canadian Paediatric Society.
www.caringforkids.cps.ca

Centre of Excellence for Early Childhood Development

Provides recommendations on the services needed to ensure the best early development in young children.
www.excellence-earlychildhood.ca

Growing Healthy Canadians

A guide for positive child development.
www.growinghealthykids.com

Immunize Canada

Information about immunizations for all ages.
www.immunize.ca

Nobody's Perfect

Offers an education and support program for parents.
www.nobodysperfect.ca

Oral Health for Children

Children's oral health care information by Health Canada.
www.hc-sc.gc.ca/hl-vs/oral-bucco/care-soin/child-enfant-eng.php

The Parent-Child Mother Goose Program

This group program uses rhymes, songs, and stories to nurture the parent-child relationship.
www.nationalpcmgp.ca

Vaccination and Your Child

Caring for kids, information for parents from the Canadian Paediatric Society. Lists the immunizations that are recommended in Canada.
www.caringforkids.cps.ca/handouts/vaccination_and_your_child

Child safety

Canadian Child Welfare Research Portal
Provides access to up-to-date research on Canadian child welfare programs and policies.
www.cwrp.ca

Car Seat Clinics in Canada
Government of Canada help to find a car seat clinic in your community.
www.canada.ca/en/services/transport/road/child-car-seat-safety/child-car-seat-clinics-other-resources.html

Car Seat Information
Ontario Government information about choosing and installing car seats.
www.mto.gov.on.ca/english/safety/choose-car-seat.shtml

Car Seat Safety
Government of Canada information about car safety for children.
www.canada.ca/en/services/transport/road/child-car-seat-safety.html

Is Your Child Safe? Series
Health Canada information on keeping young children safe from health and safety hazards.
www.hc-sc.gc.ca/cps-spc/pubs/cons/child-enfant/index-eng.php

National Center on Shaken Baby Syndrome
Find information on preventing shaken baby syndrome and how to calm an infant.
www.dontshake.org/purple-crying

Parachute
A charity helping Canadians to stop the clock on predictable and preventable injuries.
1-888-537-7777 or www.parachutecanada.org/child-injury-prevention

Prevent Child Injury
Child safety information to keep children safe and decrease child injuries.
www.preventchildinjury.ca

Safe Sleep
Information about SIDS and safe infant sleep environments.
www.publichealth.gc.ca/safesleep

Children with special needs

Your public health nurse can help if you think your baby has a developmental problem or a disability. Most communities have an infant development program for children. Staff in this program can help you with activities for your baby that will encourage development. They can also help you find support services.

Autism Canada
Works collaboratively with provincial and territorial organizations, associations, and societies to champion autism spectrum disorder priorities.
1-866-476-8440 or www.autismcanada.org

Canadian Down Syndrome Society
The Canadian Down Syndrome Society is a national non-profit organization providing information, advocacy, and education about Down syndrome. The CDSS supports self-advocates, parents, and families through all stages of life.
1-800-883-5608 or www.cdss.ca

Canadian National Institute for the Blind
Provides community-based support, knowledge, and a national voice to ensure Canadians who are blind or partially sighted have the confidence, skills, and opportunities to fully participate in life.
1-800-563-2642 or www.cnib.ca

Centre of Excellence for Children and Adolescents With Special Needs
Ensures that advanced knowledge about children and adolescents with special needs living in rural, remote, and northern locations is disseminated effectively to those who need it most.
www.specialneedsproject.ca/resources/links-directory/211-centre-of-excellence-for-children-and-adolescents-with-special-needs

Health care providers

Canadian Association of Midwives
Represents midwives and the profession of midwifery in Canada.
1-514-807-3668 or www.canadianmidwives.org

Canadian Association of Perinatal and Women's Health Nurses
Represents women's health, obstetric, and newborn nurses from across Canada.
www.capwhn.ca

Canadian Fertility and Andrology Society
Speaks on behalf of all interested parties in the field of assisted reproductive technologies and research in reproductive sciences.
1-514-524-9009 or www.cfas.ca

Canadian Nurses Association
Registered nurses contributing to the health of Canadians and the advancement of nursing.
1-800-361-8404 or www.cna-aiic.ca

College of Family Physicians of Canada
Professional organization responsible for establishing standards for the training, certification, and lifelong education of family physicians and for advocating on behalf of the specialty of family medicine, family physicians, and their patients.
1-800-387-6197 or www.cfpc.ca

Society of Obstetricians and Gynaecologists of Canada
National medical society that promotes excellence in the practice of obstetrics and gynaecology and works to advance the health of women through leadership, advocacy, collaboration, and education.
1-800-561-2416 or www.sogc.org

The Royal College of Physicians and Surgeons of Canada
Oversees the medical education of specialists in Canada. They accredit the university programs that train resident physicians for their specialty practices, and they write and administer the demanding examinations that residents must pass to become certified as specialists.
www.royalcollege.ca

Indigenous

Aboriginal Tobacco Program
The Aboriginal Tobacco Program (ATP) works with Aboriginal communities to decrease and prevent the misuse of tobacco.
www.tobaccowise.com

Beginning Journey: First Nations Pregnancy Resource
First Nations pregnancy resource by Best Start Resource Centre.
www.beststart.org/resources/rep_health/E33A_Beginning_Journey.pdf

First Nations and Inuit Health
Health Canada information on First Nations and Inuit to improve their health.
www.hc-sc.gc.ca/fniah-spnia/index-eng.php

First Nations and Inuit Health— Tobacco
Information on traditional and non-traditional use of tobacco and facts on smoking rates in First Nations and Inuit communities.
www.hc-sc.gc.ca/fniah-spnia/substan/tobac-tabac/index-eng.php

Institute of Aboriginal Peoples' Health
Fosters the advancement of a national health research agenda to improve and promote the health of First Nations, Inuit, and Métis individuals in Canada through research, knowledge translation, and capacity building.
www.cihr-irsc.gc.ca/e/8668.html

National Aboriginal Health Organization
Excels in the advancement and promotion of health and well-being of all First Nations, Inuit, and Métis individuals, families, and communities.
www.naho.ca

National Association of Friendship Centres

A network of 118 friendship centres and seven provincial and territorial associations from coast-to-coast.
www.nafc.ca

Pauktuutit: Inuit Women of Canada

Fosters a greater awareness of the needs of Inuit women and encourages their participation in community, regional, and national concerns in relation to social, cultural, and economic development.
1-800-667-0749 or www.pauktuutit.ca

Labour and birth

Caesarean birth

Information about caesarean birth from the Society of Obstetricians and Gynaecologists of Canada.
www.pregnancy.sogc.org/labour-and-childbirth/caesarean-section

Doula

Dona International provides information about what a doula is and how to find one.
www.dona.org/mothers/index.php

Induction of Labour

Induction of labour information by the MotHERS Program.
www.themothersprogram.ca/during-pregnancy/pregnancy-induction

Labour 101

Information about labour from the Society of Obstetricians and Gynaecologists of Canada.
www.pregnancy.sogc.org/labour-and-childbirth/labour-101

Preterm Labour

Information about preterm labour from the Society of Obstetricians and Gynaecologists of Canada.
www.pregnancy.sogc.org/other-considerations/preterm-labour

Vaginal Birth After Caesarean Birth

Information about vaginal birth after caesarean birth from the Society of Obstetricians and Gynaecologists of Canada.
www.pregnancy.sogc.org/labour-and-childbirth/vaginal-birth-after-caesarean-section

Vaginal Birth After Caesarean Birth

Vaginal birth after caesarean birth information by the Association of Ontario Midwives.
www.ontariomidwives.ca/images/uploads/client-resources/VBAC-final.pdf

Nutrition

Canada's Food Guide

Canada's Food Guide from Health Canada.
www.hc-sc.gc.ca/fn-an/food-guide-aliment/index-eng.php

Canada Prenatal Nutrition Program Projects Directory Online

Search for a program for pregnant women near you.
www.cpnp-pcnp.phac-aspc.gc.ca

Dietitians of Canada

Information on food and nutrition for Canadians.
www.dietitians.ca

EatRight Ontario

Get easy-to-use information on nutrition and healthy eating and speak with a registered dietitian for free. They also offer a menu planner "Eating for a Healthy Pregnancy."
1-877-510-5102 or www.eatrightontario.ca

Fish Consumption

Up-to-date warnings about fish consumption across Canada on the Government of Canada's website.
www.ec.gc.ca/mercure-mercury/default.asp?lang=En&n=DCBE5083-1

Food Safety for Pregnant Women

Offers helpful advice on how to reduce your risk of food poisoning.
www.healthycanadians.gc.ca/eating-nutrition/healthy-eating-saine-alimentation/safety-salubrite/vulnerable-populations/pregnant-enceintes-eng.php

Natural Health Products

Health Canada provides information about natural health products.
www.hc-sc.gc.ca/dhp-mps/prodnatur/about-apropos/cons-eng.php

Nutrition Guideline

"Canadian Consensus on Female Nutrition: Adolescence, Reproduction, Menopause, and Beyond" by the Society of Obstetricians and Gynaecologists of Canada.
www.jogc.com/article/ S1701-2163(16)00042-6/abstract

Nutrition Labelling

Health Canada provides nutrition labelling information.
www.hc-sc.gc.ca/fn-an/label-etiquet/nutrition/index-eng.php

Prenatal Nutrition

Health Canada provides prenatal guidelines on nutrition and healthy eating during pregnancy.
www.hc-sc.gc.ca/fn-an/nutrition/ prenatal/index_e.html

Parenting

Support programs, pregnancy outreach programs, and family resource centres offer programs and services to support families and single parents. Contact your local health office or public health nurse for more information.

Canadian Child Care Federation

Online fact sheets and resources about issues related to parenting.
1-800-858-1412 or www.cccf-fcsge.ca

Community Action Program for Children

Community Action Program for Children provides programs that address the health and development of children (0–6 years) who are living in conditions of risk.
www.capc-pace.phac-aspc.gc.ca

Multiple Births Canada

Provides support, education, research, and advocacy to individuals, families, chapters, and organizations that have a personal or professional interest in multiple birth issues.
1-866-228-8824 or www.multiplebirthscanada.org

Ontario Early Years Centres (OEYC)

These programs provide opportunities for all children to participate in play and inquiry-based programs and support all parents and caregivers in their roles. Parents and caregivers also have access to information about child development and specialized services as needed.
www.oeyc.ca

Registering a Birth in Canada

How to register a birth and apply for a birth certificate.
www.servicecanada.gc.ca/eng/ lifeevents/baby.shtml

Pregnancy

Active Pregnancy

A list of guidelines to follow before starting physical activity.
www.ophea.net/sites/default/files/ archive/resource/2010/05/parc_act ivepregnancyresourcefinal_14se09_ pdf_14027.pdf

Birth Plan

A sample birth plan is available from the Society of Obstetricians and Gynaecologists of Canada.
www.pregnancy.sogc.org/labour-and-childbirth/birth-plan

Canadian Blood Services

The Canadian Blood Services' Cord Blood Bank collects voluntarily donated cord blood units from mothers across Canada.
www.blood.ca/en/cordblood

Canadian Diabetes Association

Information about diabetes.
1-800-226-8464 or www.diabetes.ca

Canadian Human Rights Commission

Provide equal opportunity to everyone in Canada and to help people confront discrimination in their daily lives.
1-888-214-1090 or www.chrc-ccdp.ca

Cord Blood Banking
The Society of Obstetricians and Gynaecologists of Canada offers information on cord blood banking.
www.pregnancy.sogc.org/labour-and-childbirth/umbilical-cord-blood

Due Date Calculator
Due date calculator by the Society of Obstetricians and Gynaecologists of Canada.
www.pregnancy.sogc.org/due-date-calculator

Health Before Pregnancy
The Best Start Resource Centre's website offers information about health before pregnancy.
www.healthbeforepregnancy.ca

Healthy Pregnancy
Government of Canada information about a healthy pregnancy.
www.healthycanadians.gc.ca/healthy-living-vie-saine/pregnancy-grossesse/index-eng.php?

Héma-Québec
Public cord blood bank in Québec.
www.hema-quebec.qc.ca

Motherisk
Information and guidance for pregnant or breastfeeding women about risks associated with drug, chemical, infection, disease, and radiation exposures.
Motherisk helpline: 1-877-439-2744
Alcohol and substance:
1-877-327-4636
Morning sickness: 1-800-436-8477
www.motherisk.org

Nausea and Vomiting During Pregnancy
The Society of Obstetricians and Gynaecologists of Canada offers information on nausea and vomiting during pregnancy.
www.pregnancy.sogc.org/nausea-and-vomiting-in-pregnancy

OMama
OMama connects women and families to trusted, evidence-informed healthy pregnancy, birth, and early parenting information for Ontario.
www.omama.com

Oral Health During Pregnancy
Government of Canada information about oral health during pregnancy.
www.healthycanadians.gc.ca/healthy-living-vie-saine/pregnancy-grossesse/general-information-renseignements-generaux/oral-buccodentaire-eng.php?

Ovulation Calculator—Baby Center
Online tool for figuring out when you are likely ovulating.
www.babycenter.ca/ovulation-calculator

Policy on Pregnancy and Human Rights in the Workplace
The Canadian Human Rights Commission Policy on Pregnancy and Human Rights in the Workplace.
www.chrc-ccdp.gc.ca/eng/content/policy-and-best-practices-page-1

Pregnancy
Information about pregnancy and childbirth from the Society of Obstetricians and Gynaecologists of Canada.
www.pregnancy.sogc.org

Pregnancy Leave and Parental Leave
Government of Canada information about pregnancy leave and parental leaves.
www.servicecanada.gc.ca/eng/lifeevents/baby.shtml

Public Health Agency of Canada—Healthy Pregnancy
Public Health Agency of Canada information on healthy pregnancy.
www.phac-aspc.gc.ca/hp-gs/think-pense-eng.php

The Sensible Guide to a Healthy Pregnancy
A guide to help you to make good decisions about how to take care of yourself before, during, and after your pregnancy.
www.phac-aspc.gc.ca/hp-gs/guide/ index-eng.php

Ultrasound in Pregnancy
The Society of Obstetricians and Gynaecologists of Canada offers information on ultrasound in pregnancy.
www.pregnancy.sogc.org/routine- tests/ultrasound-in-pregnancy

Women's Health Matters Pregnancy Health Centre
Online information about pregnancy.
www.womenshealthmatters.ca/ health-centres/sexual-health/ pregnancy

Postpartum depression

Canadian Mental Health Association: Postpartum Depression
Information about postpartum depression.
www.cmha.ca/mental_health/ postpartum-depression

Emotional Health in Pregnancy
Public Health Agency of Canada information on emotional health in pregnancy.
www.phac-aspc.gc.ca/hp-gs/ guide/07_eh-se-eng.php

Mental Health During Pregnancy and with a New Baby
Provides pregnant women and new parents with information on mental health during pregnancy, the baby blues and postpartum mood disorders.
http://en.beststart.org/for_parents/ are-you-or-your-partner-pregnant

Mood Disorders Society of Canada
Postpartum depression information.
www.mdcs.ca

Sexual health

Action Canada for Sexual Health and Rights
Information and resources on sexual and reproductive health.
1-888-642-2725 or www.sexualhealthandrights.ca

Canadian Fertility and Andrology Society
Speaks on behalf of all interested parties in the field of assisted reproductive technologies and research in reproductive sciences.
www.cfas.ca

HIV and AIDS
Government of Canada's information about HIV and AIDS.
www.healthycanadians.gc.ca/ diseases-conditions-maladies- affections/disease-maladie/hiv- aids-vih-sida/index-eng.php

Infertility Awareness Association of Canada
National organization providing educational material, support, and assistance to individuals and couples who are experiencing the anguish of infertility.
1-800-263-2929 or www.fertilitymatters.ca

SexandU.ca
The Society of Obstetricians and Gynaecologists of Canada's website provides Canada's one-stop source for information on sexual and reproductive health, contraception, and sexually transmitted infections.
www.sexandu.ca

Smoking cessation

Canadian Cancer Society—Smokers' Helpline
Free, confidential service operated by the Canadian Cancer Society offering support and information about quitting smoking and tobacco use.
1-877-513-5333 or www.smokershelpline.ca

Pregnets—Smoking and Pregnancy
Improves the health of moms and their babies by offering information, resources, and support to pregnant and postpartum women and their health care providers.
www.pregnets.org

Quit Now
*Online resource and telephone
support for people who want to quit
smoking. They help you design your
individual quit plan while offering
support by texts and through their
24-hour-per-day call-in number.
1-877-455-2233 or www.quitnow.ca*

Tobacco
*Health Canada's tobacco website
provides a comprehensive range
of information and resources on
tobacco control.
www.hc-sc.gc.ca/hc-ps/tobac-tabac/
index-eng.php*

Other reading

The Canadian Paediatric Society Guide to Caring for Your Child From Birth to Age Five (2009)
Author: Diane Sacks. Publisher: The Canadian Paediatric Society.

This book is the complete parenting guide from Canada's leading child and youth health care experts. Focusing on health, growth and development, safety, nutrition, and with a special section dedicated to emotional well-being, this book gives you the answers you need from the organization that doctors and parents have relied on for decades.

Your Child's Best Shot: A Parent's Guide to Vaccination (2015)
Author: Dr. Dorothy L. Moore. Publisher: The Canadian Paediatric Society.

With so much information on immunization available from conflicting and often questionable sources, it's easy to get overwhelmed or confused about the facts. *Your Child's Best Shot* is the only comprehensive Canadian reference written specifically for parents.

Your Baby and Child: From Birth to Age Five (2010)
Author: Penelope Leach. Publisher: Alfred A. Knopf, New York

This newest edition of Penelope Leach's much-loved, trusted, and comprehensive classic—an international best-seller for 25 years, with nearly two million copies sold in America alone—encompasses the latest research and thinking on child development and learning, reflecting the realities of today's changing lifestyles.

Dr. Jack Newman's Guide to Breastfeeding (2014)
Authors: Dr. Jack Newman and Teresa Pitman. Publisher: HarperCollins Canada.

This book was written by Dr. Jack Newman, a paediatrician, and Teresa Pitman, a Canadian expert on breastfeeding and international board-certified lactation consultant. It offers extensive practical information and encouragement on breastfeeding.

Use the space provided on page 252 to write down all the important contact information you will need before you go into labour. Once it's time to go to the hospital, you won't need to scramble and you can follow the following action list.

You are in labour and it's time to go the hospital when:

- Your water breaks in a gush or is leaking steadily.
- Your contractions are regular and 5 minutes apart (and the hospital or birth centre is LESS than 30 minutes away).
- Your contractions are regular and 10 minutes apart (and the hospital or birth centre is MORE than 30 minutes away).

NOTE: If you don't know how to measure your contractions (see page 147), or if you are still unsure, *you should contact or see a health care provider.*

What to do when you go into labour:

Action List

- ☐ Call your ride, the ambulance, or a taxi.
- ☐ Call your labour support team: partner, labour coach, and/or whoever you would like with you at the hospital or birthing centre.
- ☐ Call your babysitter and pet sitter to arrange for care while you're in the hospital or birthing centre (if needed).
- ☐ Grab your suitcase (refer to page 138 for recommended items for you and your baby). Don't forget taxi or parking money.
- ☐ Celebrate! Call your family members and friends.

Contact list

Transportation

Ambulance: Phone:

Ride to hospital: Phone: Cell:

Alternate ride to hospital: Phone: Cell:

Taxi: Phone:

Labour support

Partner: Phone: Cell:

Labour coach: Phone: Cell:

Support network

Babysitter: Phone: Cell:

Pet sitter: Phone: Cell:

Household help: Phone: Cell:

Neighbour: Phone: Cell:

Public health nurse: Phone: Cell:

Breastfeeding consultant: Phone: Cell:

Family and friends

Name: Phone: Cell:

Name: Phone: Cell:

Name: Phone: Cell:

Medical contacts

Health care provider: Phone: Cell:

Health care provider: Phone: Cell:

Paediatrician: Phone: Cell:

Hospital or birthing center address:

Hospital or birthing centre   Phone:

List of appointments with my health care providers

Health care provider name   **Date/Time**

Index

A

abdomen
    menstrual cycle discomfort, 15
    muscles in, 189
    surgery, 96
abuse (violence), 240
    digital, 82
    emotional, 81, 101
    financial, 82
    physical, 81, 101
    during pregnancy, 80
    preterm labour and, 101
    sexual, 81
    spiritual, 82
    types of, 81–82
    verbal, 81
accidents, 96
acne, baby, 216
acquired immune deficiency syndrome (AIDS), 70–71
active stage, of labour, 152
    coping with, 156
acupressure, 72
acupuncture treatment, 72
aerobic exercise, 55–56
    rules to follow, 57
after-pains, 187–188
aging placenta, 139, 141
AIDS. See acquired immune deficiency syndrome
alcohol, 240–241
    avoidance of, 23
    FASD, 37
    harmful effects of, 36
    quiz on, 36
amniocentesis, 65, 66
anaesthetics. See freezing medicines
analgesics. See painkillers
anemia
    iron and, 30
    risk for, 30
antibodies, blood type and, 60, 63
Apgar score, 168–169
artificial sweeteners, avoidance of, 24
assisted births, 171–172
augmenting labour, 118–119

B

baby. See also newborns; overdue babies
    acne, 216
    bonding with, 167–168, 200
    breech, 170–171
    death of, 176–178
    feeding, 219–220
    first check-up, 204
    first impression of, 198–199
    full term, 137–138
    growth measurement of, 88, 137
    handling of, 199–200
    health care provider and, 204–205
    health problems of, 176–177
    herpes risk, 69
    hormones and sex organs of, 199
    immunization and, 205–206
    jaundice and, 207–209
    journal for, 179
    laboratory testing for health of, 62–63
    language and, 200
    monitoring of, 119, 150, 151
    preterm, 102–103
    second-hand screens and, 200–201
    water for, 125, 126, 130
baby blues. See postpartum depression
baby safety
    car seats, 202–203
    diaper changes, 213
    in home, 201
    around other people, 202
    outdoors, 202
backaches, 92
    exercise for, 59
    during labour, 159
    preterm labour and, 100
bathing, of newborns, 213–214
bereavement (grief), 177–178, 241
bilirubin, 207
birth, 243–244
    after, 166–168
    action list for, 251
    assisted, 171–172
    body changes after, 182–183
    discomforts after giving, 186–188
    emotions after, 176–177
    expectations during, 114–115
    follow-up home care, 175–176
    hospital stay after, 174–176
    journal for after, 195
    positions for, 120
    suction-assisted, 172
    to-do list after, 180, 196
birth canal, 157–158, 170–171, 199
birth centre. See family-centred care checklist; hospitals
birth control, 186, 190–194
    breastfeeding and, 191
    condoms, 192
    diaphragms or cervical caps, 192
    forms of, 16–17, 193
    IUD, 192
    patch, 16, 191
    pill, 16, 191
    ring, 16, 191
    shot, 16, 191–192
    spermicides, 192
    sterilization, 194
birth defects, 30
    genetic disorders and, 61
    risk of, 61
birth plan
    common things to include, 117
    discussion of, 116–117
    need for, 116
    religious or cultural beliefs, 121
    writing of, 116
birth preparation, 51–52
birthing team, 149
bladder infections, 98–99
bleeding. See also hemorrhage, postpartum; light bleeding; vaginal discharge
    caesarean birth and, 173
    during second trimester, 96
    unusual, 185
blocked milk ducts, 230
blood testing, 60
    during labour, 118
blood type, antibodies and, 60, 63
bloody show, 147